Phone Numbers

School name, phone: _____

Teacher's name, phone: _____

School counselor name, phone: _____

School name, phone: _____

Teacher's name, phone: _____

School counselor name, phone: _____

Coach's name, phone: _____

Coach's name, phone: _____

Clubs or groups for teens:

Name: _____ Phone: _____

Name: _____ Phone: _____

Name: _____ Phone: _____

Name: _____ Phone: _____

Teen's friends:

Name: _____ Phone: _____

Name: _____ Phone: _____

Name: _____ Phone: _____

Name: _____ Phone: _____

Other phone numbers:

Name: _____ Phone: _____

Name: _____ Phone: _____

Name: _____ Phone: _____

Name: _____ Phone: _____

What To Do For Teen Health

Easy to Read • Easy to Use

Gloria Mayer, R.N.
Ann Kuklierus, R.N.

Institute for Healthcare Advancement
501 S. Idaho St., Suite 300
La Habra, California 90631
(800) 434-4633

© 2008 Institute for Healthcare Advancement
501 S. Idaho Street, Suite 300
La Habra, California 90631
(800) 434-4633

Printed in the United States
10 09 08   6 5 4
ISBN: 978-0-9701245-2-4

To Our Readers

This book is for moms, dads, and others who have teens. It explains the body changes that happen to teens. It will help you explain these changes to your teen.

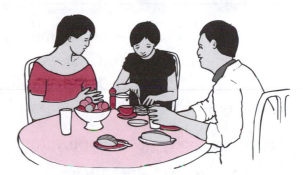

This book gives you tips on how to deal with teen issues such as dating, school, driving, smoking, and drugs. It will help you talk with your teen about these things.

This book tells you about the signs of trouble and where to get help. It will help you understand the teen years and know what to do to keep your teen safe and healthy.

Here are some things to do when you get this book.

- Fill in the phone numbers in the front of the book. Keep this book where it is easy to find.

- Turn to page viii to find out what's in this book.

- See page vii to learn when you should get help for your teen. Read pages 33–35 for a list of people and places for help with your teen.

- Read a few pages of this book every day until you have read it all.

- See the word list at the end of the book. It gives the meaning of certain words in the book.

To Our Readers

This book was read by doctors and others who work with teens. They agree with the information in this book. They feel it is safe and helpful.

But each teen is different. Some things in this book may not be right for your teen. You must decide what to do and when to get help. If you are worried about your teen or have questions about anything in this book, get help right away.

There are many people you can go to for help such as:

- Doctors and nurses
- School teachers and counselors
- Social workers
- Priests, ministers, and rabbis
- Hotlines and support groups

Always do what your doctor or other trained person tells you.

When to Get Help For Your Teen

Your teen is changing. It is hard to know what is normal and what is not. Get help if your teen:

- Talks about dying.
- Is giving things away.
- Is mean to animals.
- Takes drugs or gets drunk.
- Was raped.
- Is losing or gaining a lot of weight.
- Looks sick.
- Is always tired.
- Fights with everyone.
- Threatens to run away.
- Seems angry all the time.
- Is failing in school.
- Is in trouble with the law.
- Spends all his time alone.
- Has no friends.
- Comes and goes without talking to anyone in the family.
- May be pregnant.
- Had unprotected sex.
- Is on drugs.

Read this book for more signs of when to get help for your teen.

What's in This Book

What's in This Book

The Teen Years: A Time of Big Changes

Notes

_____

_____

_____

_____

_____

_____

_____

_____

_____

_____

_____

_____

_____

Emotions

What is it?

Emotions are very strong feelings. A teen's emotions can change very fast. Teens may be happy one minute and sad the next.

Did you know?

- As your children become teens, their needs change. Your role as a mom or dad may change also. This is normal.

- Teens can cry, laugh, or get angry all in a short time. This is called mood swings. Mood swings are normal. They come from changes in the hormones (body juices) of growing boys and girls.

- Teens often don't know what they feel or want. They don't know why they are sad. Talking about feelings can help teens learn what is wrong.

- Teens love and hate their parents at the same time. This is normal. They want to be left alone. At the same time, they want help from their parents.

- Anger is an emotion. It can be a sign of a problem.

- Actions and emotions are different among teens. This is normal.

- Teens worry about many things. They worry about:
  - School grades
  - Money
  - Not having enough time
  - What other people think of them
  - Their future
- Teens may not seem to care about things, but they care very much.

What can I do?

- Tell your teen that the body changes affect how he or she feels. This is normal.

- Praise your teen for doing things right.

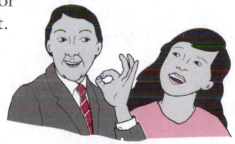

- Accept your teen. Never make fun of him or her. Don't tease your teen.

- Teens often copy what others do. Set a good example for what you want your teen to do.

- Talk with your teen about feelings. Watch for signs of anger. If you don't help your teen with anger, bad things can happen. Read about anger on page 60.

- Spend time with your teen. Listen to what your teen says even if you don't agree. Don't tell your teen what he or she says is good or bad. Just let your teen talk about things.

Emotions

- Tell the family, including brothers and sisters, not to fight with the teen. If your teen acts badly, she should be left alone.

- Know what your teen does every day. Meet your teen's friends.

- Make sure punishment fits your teen's actions. Don't over punish your teen for something small. Don't let your teen talk you out of punishment.

- Pick your fights. Don't fight over small things.

- Set limits for your teen. Also tell your teen important things he or she needs to do.

- Let your teen have his or her way when possible. Even if you don't like what your teen wears, it might be OK to let him or her wear it. This lets teens have their way about safe things.

- Try to include your teen in family time but don't force him.

- Be honest and show respect for your teen. Listen to your teen. Don't accuse your teen of anything without having all the facts.

- Don't lecture or talk **at** your teen. Discuss things with your teen.

When should I get help?

- Your teen talks about killing him or herself.
- Your teen has been abused.
- Your teen throws up after eating, is not eating, or is losing a lot of weight.
- You think your teen is taking drugs, drinking alcohol, or is breaking the law.
- Your teen has no friends. He or she spends most of the time alone.
- You are very mad at your teen. You feel like hurting your teen.
- Your teen is not going to school or is getting poor grades.
- Your teen has a gun or knife.
- Your teen talks about hurting another person.
- Your teen is mean to animals.

Body Changes in Boys

What is it?

During the teen years a boy's body changes from a child to an adult. This time of fast growth is called puberty. These body changes allow boys to make babies.

Did you know?

- Changes can start in boys as early as 8 years old or as late as 15. Changes take 3–5 years.
- Here is a list of the changes that happen:
  - Fine, straight hairs start to grow around the penis.
  - The testicles (also called balls) and the sac they are in (scrotum) grow bigger.
  - The penis grows wider and longer.
  - The voice starts to change.
  - Hairs start to grow on the upper lip.
  - Hair grows under the arms and on the face.
  - The hair around the penis gets dark and thick.
  - The boy grows taller.

Body Changes in Boys

Here are pictures showing how a boy's body changes.

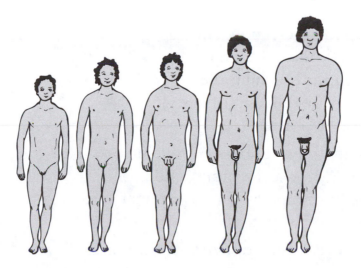

- Boys grow tall in the later teen years. A boy is tall like an adult by age 18.

- Boys get strong during this time and look lean.

- A boy's voice gets deeper during this time. A boy's voice may crack while talking. This is normal.

- Boys start to ejaculate semen during the night. This is called a wet dream. There is nothing a boy can do to stop this. It is normal. Wet dreams happen less often after a boy is done with body changes.

- A boy can get a girl pregnant once he has semen. This happens between 11 and 17 years old.

7

Body Changes in Boys

- A boy's penis may become hard at any time. This is called an erection. An erection can happen without touching the penis or thinking of sex. This is normal.

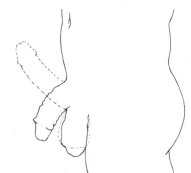

- Some boys' breasts get bigger. They may feel a bump under one or both nipples. This is normal and will go away.

- Uneven balls (testicles) are normal.

- Some boys are circumcised. This means the skin over the tip of the penis (foreskin) is cut off. The penis looks different if the foreskin is gone. Both ways are normal.

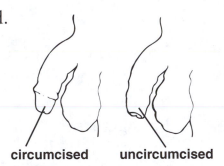

circumcised   uncircumcised

- A boy's body starts to smell at this time. Boys need to take showers every day and put deodorant under their arms.

What can I do?

- Talk with your teen about body changes. Do this before the changes start.

- Tell your teen the changes are normal.

- Show your teen pictures like the ones in this book. Let him ask questions.

Body Changes in Boys

- Explain wet dreams and erections. Tell your teen that it may make him blush or feel shy. Give him ideas on how to hide an erection like wearing big shirts and pants.

- Talk about washing the penis. If he is not circumcised, tell your teen to pull back the foreskin when washing the penis and then return it to its position.

- Talk about body smell and what to do about it.

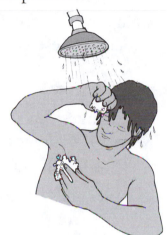

- Your teen needs to know how babies are made by this time.

- Don't make fun of your teen's body changes. Teens worry about what people say about their body.

When should I get help?

- Teen has pain in his groin or sex parts.

- Teen can't pull back the foreskin to wash the penis.

- Your teen is having sex.

- Your teen has pain when peeing (passing urine).

- Teen is a lot shorter than his friends.

- Pus is coming out of the penis.

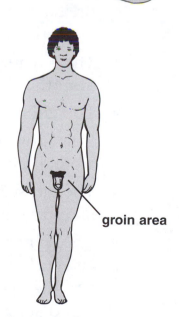

groin area

Body Changes in Girls

What is it?

During the teen years a girl's body changes from a child to an adult. This time of fast growth is called puberty. These changes allow girls to have babies.

Did you know?

- Changes can start in girls as early as 8 years or as late as 14. Changes can last for 4–5 years.
- Here's a list of the body changes that happen:
  - Hairs start to grow around the lips of the vagina.
  - Breasts begin to grow. At first they look like little bumps under the nipples.
  - The red area around the nipples grows out from the chest.
  - The girl grows taller.
  - Hair grows on the legs, under the arms, and around the genitals.
  - The girl starts having periods. This is called menstruation.
  - The hair around the genitals gets dark and curly.
  - The breasts grow to their full size and shape.

Body Changes in Girls

Here are pictures showing how a girl's body changes.

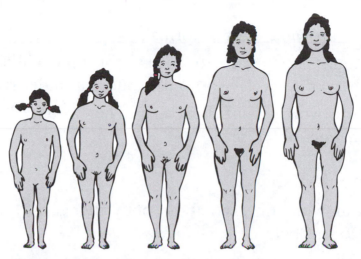

- Girls grow tall during the early teen years. They stop growing at around age 16.

- Girls gain weight during this time. They need to gain a certain amount of weight to start having periods. This does not mean that girls get fat.

- Periods can start between 10 and 14 years of age. Most girls get their period around 12–13 years old.

- Fluid leaks from the vagina before the period starts. The fluid can be clear or white. It can be watery or thick. This is normal.

- At first, periods are not regular. A teen can skip a month. Periods last from 2–5 days.

- At first a girl may have no pain with her period. Later she may have cramps the first few days. Motrin or other over-the-counter medicines help the pain.

- One breast may grow bigger than the other. The small one will catch up. The breasts may be sore while they are growing. This is normal.

- A girl's body starts to smell at this time. Girls need to shower every day and put deodorant under their arms.

- Girls worry about their body. They wonder if these changes are normal.

What can I do?

- Talk with your teen about body changes. Do this before the changes start.

- Tell your teen the changes are normal.

- Show your teen pictures like the ones in this book.

- Have a private talk with your teen. Talk about breast and hair growth, periods, and other things. Tell your teen about normal vaginal fluid.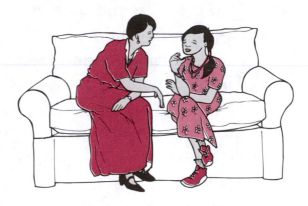

- Teach your teen what to do when she gets her period. This is very important. She needs to know this before she gets her first period.

- Show her what she will need to use for her period such as pads and tampons. Make sure she can get them at school or carries them with her.

Body Changes in Girls

- Talk with your teen about body smells and what to do. Your teen will need to shower or bathe every day.

- Do something nice with your teen the day she has her first period.

- Don't say bad things about periods or breast growth. Don't call it a "curse" or use other bad names.

- Tell your teen about ovulation. It is when an egg comes out of the ovary and goes into the uterus.

- Before your teen has her first period she should know how babies are made.

- Don't make fun of your teen's body changes. Girls worry about what people say about their body.

- Listen to your teen's feelings about growing up. She may fear leaving her childhood behind.

When should I get help?

- Teen has not had a period by age 14.

- Teen has a lot of pain with her periods. The pain does not go away after taking Motrin or other over-the-counter medicines.

- Teen is having sex.

- Teen is much shorter than her friends.

- Your teen has fluid coming out of the vagina that does not seem normal.

How Parents Can Help Teens

Notes

_____

_____

_____

_____

_____

_____

_____

_____

_____

_____

_____

_____

_____

_____

Building Self-Esteem

What is it?

Self-esteem is how a person feels about him or herself. It is the feeling of worth or value.

Did you know?

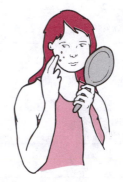

- The teen years are hard on self-esteem. Body changes make teens feel insecure. Teens worry about how they look.

- Teens are unsure about who they are.

- Parents and friends help shape a teen's self-esteem.

- Saying nice things to a teen helps build self-esteem.

- Doing well in school, sports, or other things builds self-esteem.

- Teens with high self-esteem make good choices.

- Teens with low self-esteem are not happy. They feel that they are not good enough.

- Teens who don't feel good about themselves don't take care of their bodies. They try to feel better by doing things like smoking, taking drugs, and drinking alcohol. They may have sex to feel loved.

- Low self-esteem is bad for a teen's health.

Building Self-Esteem

What can I do?

- Build strong self-esteem in your teen. Help your teen feel good. Here are some things you can do:
  - Praise your teen often, but be honest.
  - Brag about your teen and let him or her hear you.
  - Help your teen find things that he or she is good at. Your teen may be good at music, sports, or art.
  - Tell your teen often that you are proud.
- Don't call your teen names such as "stupid." Don't put your teen down.
- Don't pick on small things. Don't look for reasons to correct your teen. Look for reasons to praise your teen.
- Celebrate your teen's successes. Treat your teen to something special when he or she does well on a test.
- Tell your teen often that you love him or her. Put notes in your teen's bag or other places where your teen will find them. Here are some things you can write:
  - I'm thinking about you.
  - You can do it!
  - You are terrific!
  - You are special!
  - Good luck on your test.
  - I'm proud of you.
  - Here's a hug. Have a great day!

- Friends can help or hurt your teen's self-esteem. Help your teen pick good friends. Talk with your teen about what makes a good friend. Read about friends on page 38.

When should I get help?

- Your teen always puts herself down.
- Your teen will not try new things.
- Your teen is always afraid of failing.
- Your teen spends most of the time alone.
- You are worried about your teen.
- Your teen has lost interest in things he or she used to like.

Family Time

What is it?

Family time is when everyone in the family gets together to do something.

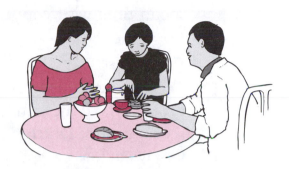

Did you know?

- Teens who are close to their family have fewer problems with drugs and the law. The family teaches teens values. It teaches them how to get along with others.

- The teen years are full of hard times. Teens need the support of their family when they are sad or worried.

- Teens act like they don't want to be part of the family. They think it's not cool to be seen with parents.

- Teens often feel like little children when they are with their parents. So they may set rules such as:

  - No hugs or kisses in public.

  - They want to be dropped off at the corner.

  - They don't want to be seen with their parents.

- Teens love their parents. They just don't show it. Friends and outside activities become more important than family. This is normal.

- Parents must slowly let go of their teen. Letting go can be hard for parents.

What can I do?

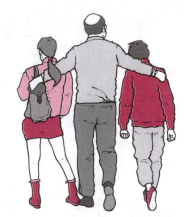

- The best thing you can do is spend time with your teen. Look for ways to stay close to your teen.

- Teens need to feel part of a group. Make the family your teen's group. Do things as a family such as camping or hiking.

- Start a family project such as planting a garden. Take up a family sport.

- Give your teen some power in the family. Let your teen make choices. This will make your teen feel good. Let your teen choose:
  - Where to go out to eat.
  - What to have for dinner.
  - Which movie to see.

- Eat several meals a week as a family. It can be hard to get everyone together, but it is important. It is a good time to stay in touch with your teen. Turn the TV off. It's a time for the family to talk and laugh together.

- Have your teen help with the meal and the cleanup.

- Plan things to do as a family. If your teen does not want to join in, ask if he would like to bring a friend.

- Kids in a family often fight. It is best to let them work things out themselves. Don't take sides. Set rules such as no hitting.

- Don't let your teen have a TV or computer in his room. Your teen will spend too much time alone. Keep the TV and computer in the family area. This will help your teen spend more time with the family. You will also be able to keep an eye on what your teen is watching and doing.

- Give your teen jobs to do as a member of the family. Some things your teen can do are:
  - Wash the family car.
  - Take out the trash.
  - Wash the dishes.
  - Keep his or her room tidy.

- Set aside one night a week as family night.
  Do something together as a family on that night.

- Do things alone with your teen like shopping or having lunch.

- If your family is religious, go to church or temple together.

When should I get help?

- Your teen is never at home.
- Your teen refuses to be part of the family.
- Your teen feels like a stranger to you.
- You can't talk with your teen.

Love and Understanding

What is it?

It is seeing good things in your teen all the time.

Did you know?

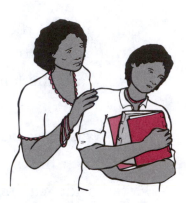

- Teens need love and understanding from parents.
- They need to feel hope. They need to know that:
  - The teen years will pass.
  - Everything will be OK.
  - One day they will be happy adults.
  - They have a good future.
- Teens who get love and understanding at home are less likely to break the law. They don't need to find love and support in gangs.

What can I do?

- Read about the changes that happen to teens (see pages 2–13). This will help you understand why your teen acts the way he or she does.
- Love and accept your teen. The teen years will pass. It may feel like forever right now. Soon your teen will grow up and move away.

Love and Understanding

- The love and understanding you show your teen today will build a strong bond for the future.

- Talk with your teen about how hard the teen years are. Tell your teen about problems and fears you had when you were a teen. This will show your teen you understand.

- Look for the good in your teen all the time.

- Before you get upset about something ask yourself "How big a deal is this?" Save yourself for the really big things like drugs.

- Your teen will make mistakes. Learn to overlook some things. Don't pick on your teen for everything.

- Say nice things to your teen. Talk about the things you like about your teen. Tell your teen what he or she does well.

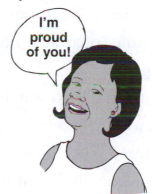

I'm proud of you!

When should I get help?

- You can't talk with your teen.
- Your teen will not let you get close to him or her.
- You don't feel love toward your teen.
- You and your teen always fight.

Rules and Discipline

What is it?

Rules are limits put on teens' actions. Rules are also things teens need to do. Discipline is what happens when teens break a rule or do something wrong.

Did you know?

- Teens need some rules or limits. It helps teens feel secure. It helps them know what is right.
- Parents set rules for things such as:
  - What time to come home at night (curfew)
  - Dating
  - How much TV to watch
  - Homework
  - Driving
  - Smoking, alcohol, and drugs
  - Chores at home
  - Telling the truth
- Teens should not have too many rules. The rules should be fair.
- The rules need to be the same when parents are in a good mood or a bad one. This makes teens feel secure. They know how to act and what to expect.
- Teens need to know what will happen if they break the rules.

Rules and Discipline

- Teens like to test the rules. This is normal.

- Discipline teaches teens what is right. It also keeps them safe. Punishment is a form of discipline.

- The most common disciplines for teens are:
  - Taking away things like the use of the phone, TV, or car.
  - Not allowing a teen to go out. This is called grounding.
  - Taking away a teen's allowance.

- Discipline should not be too hard. It should be fair. For example, if a teen comes home 30 minutes late from a date it may be unfair to ground her for a month.

- Discipline used on young children doesn't work for teens. Sending a teen to her room is not punishment. It's where a teen wants to be.

What can I do?

- Set family rules. Tell your teen what you expect.

- Set clear rules. Don't say, "Be home early." This is not clear. Say, "Be home by 10PM."

- Don't make too many rules. Teens need to start making their own choices.

- Be fair. Think about your discipline. Don't punish your teen when you are angry. You may punish too hard.

- Your teen is watching and learning from you. Make sure your teen learns the right things.

Rules and Discipline

- Next time your teen breaks a rule, ask your teen what you should do. You may be surprised by what your teen says.

- Don't look for reasons to correct your teen. Look for reasons to praise your teen. Think back on what you said to your teen today. Did you say any nice things to your teen?

- Discipline your teen out of love, not anger. Your teen will make you very angry at times. Stay calm. Don't lose your cool! Take deep breaths before you speak or act.

- Never hit your teen. This will start a pattern of violence. Control yourself, no matter how angry you are. If you think you may lose control, walk away.

- If you lose control, tell your teen you are sorry. You made a mistake. Your teen will respect you. It will teach your teen what to do when he or she makes a mistake.

- Make sure your teen feels loved, even when your teen did something wrong. Tell your teen you are upset with what he did, but you still love him.

- Hug your teen every day.

- Make sure your teen knows he can always come to you for help.

- When your teen comes to you, don't yell or get angry. Stay calm. Teach by your example how to listen and fix a problem.

- Don't try to fix everything. Stand by and let your teen solve some problems.

- Help your teen learn from mistakes. Ask your teen these questions to help him or her learn.
  - What did you learn?
  - What can you do to make things right?
  - What can you do to avoid the problem in the future?
- Teach your teen that there are small mistakes and big mistakes in life. Small mistakes are ones we can fix such as:
  - Failing a test.
  - Coming home late.
  - Missing sports practice.
- Big mistakes are ones that hurt and limit a teen's life forever. An example of a big mistake is breaking the law, using drugs, or getting pregnant. Teach your teen to think before doing something. Is he or she making a big mistake?
- Don't be too hard on your teen if he or she makes a small mistake. Your teen may get angry and fight back. Or, your teen may be afraid to come to you next time.
- Don't try to control your teen's every action. This may make your teen angry. Teens need to make some choices and mistakes. This helps them learn.
- Show by your actions that you trust and respect your teen.
- Don't forget to praise your teen for following the rules. Say things like:
  - I noticed you came home on time last night. I'm proud of you.
  - You did a good job cleaning your room. It looks very nice.

When should I get help?

- Your teen is getting into trouble with the law.
- Your teen refuses to follow the family rules.
- You can't control your anger or your temper.
- You are hitting your teen.
- Your teen is hitting you.
- Your teen lies all the time.
- Your teen is using drugs.

Talking with Your Teen

What is it?

Talking with your teen lets your teen know he or she is loved. Talking is the way to stay close to your teen. It's how you learn about your teen's feelings, fears, and dreams.

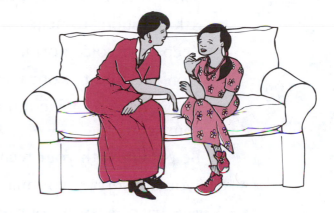

Did you know?

- It's very important for parents to talk with their teens.
- Talking with teens can be hard. It often ends in yelling.
- How teens react to parents depends on:
  - The words said.
  - The tone of voice.
  - The look on the parent's face.

What can I do?

- Use any free time to talk with your teen. A good time to talk is when you and your teen are in the car.
- Don't tell your teen that her problems are small.

Talking with Your Teen

- Talk with your teen the way you would like your teen to talk with you. Here are some things you can do:

    - Stop what you are doing.

    - Listen to your teen. Your teen will listen to you better if first you listen to your teen.

    - Ask questions to help you understand.

    - Keep your voice normal.

    - Don't lecture to your teen.

    - Don't tease or make fun of your teen.

    - Be patient with your teen.

- Say you are sorry if you make a mistake.

- Always try to answer your teen's questions. Tell your teen if you don't know the answer. Then, find the answer together.

Here are two examples of a parent and teen talking. Note how the teen reacts to what the parent says.

The **wrong** way to talk with your teen:

Teen: See you later.

Parent: Just where do you think you're going?

Teen: Out!

Parent: No, you're not! You know the rules. Since you failed your math test, you're not going out all week.

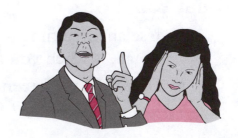

Talking with Your Teen

Teen: But I'm going to Tom's house to work on math.

Parent: No way. He dropped out of school. He's a bum who does nothing all day. He's trying to get you into trouble.

Teen: That's not true! You just don't like him.

Parent: What's there to like? Just look at him, shaved head, ring in the nose, and tattoo on his arm. He's a bum!

Teen: You don't like any of my friends! Sometimes I wonder if you like me!

Parent: That's enough stupid talk. Go to your room and do your homework!

Teen: You can't tell me what to do! I'm going out.

Parent: If you walk out that door don't bother coming back!

Teen: Fine, I'll just stay at Tom's!

The **right** way to talk with your teen:

Teen: See you later.

Parent: It's a school night. Where are you going?

Teen: I'm going to Tom's to study.

Parent: Is there something I can help you with?

Teen: No, I just need a break.

Parent: You have been working hard and I'm proud of you. But we agreed that you would not go out until you catch up on your homework.

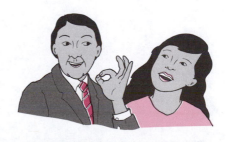

Teen: I know, but I need a break.

Parent: If you need a break, why don't we go for a walk around the block together?

Teen: No thanks, I think I'll just go back to my room.

When should I get help?

- Your teen refuses to talk with you.
- You and your teen can't talk without yelling.
- You are worried about your teen.

Getting Help for Your Teen

What is it?

Some problems are too big for parents to handle alone. They need to get help from people trained in teen problems.

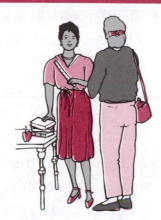

Did you know?

- The teen years are hard on everyone in the family. There are many places parents can go for help.

- Talking with other parents of teens helps. Parents don't feel so alone when they know other parents have the same problems.

- Hospitals, churches, mosques, or temples, schools, and the YMCA often have parenting classes.

  - These are good places to meet other parents who have the same concerns.

  - The classes are given by experts on teen issues.

  - They give parents ideas about what to do.

  - They help parents find other places to go for help.

What can I do?

- Your teen is changing. Sometimes you may feel you don't know your own child. It's hard to know what is normal and what is not. Talk with someone if you are worried about your teen. Don't wait. Do it right away.

Getting Help for Your Teen

- Talk with your teen's doctor if you are worried about your teen. The doctor can tell you the right thing to do.

- Your teen's school is a good place to go for help. Teachers and counselors know a lot about teens. They know if things your teen is doing are normal.

- Many schools have a list of places to call if your teen is having problems with drugs, alcohol, or smoking. Get the list. Call and ask for help.

- Get your teen to join a youth group from a church, mosque, temple, or other reliable place. Your teen will be busy, safe, and will make new friends.

- Ask your religious leader to talk with your teen.

- Look for the Social Service Resource Directory at your teen's school or in the library. It explains problems and tells you where to get help.

- Call the national hotlines or ask your teen to call.

- Two places to call are the National Youth Crisis Hotline at 1-800-448-4663 or the National Adolescent Suicide Hotline at 1-800-621-4000. These calls are free.

- Look in the front of your phone book for places to call in your area for help.

- Find the YMCA or a boys and girls club in your area. These are good places for your teen to join for social activities.

- You and your teen may need to talk with a social worker. There are different kinds of social workers. Some work only with teens. They know about the problems teens have, like drugs and alcohol.

They can help your teen. They can send you to the right place for help. Get the name of a social worker in your area from your doctor, the school, or your health plan.

- Don't be afraid to ask for help. You are not a bad parent. Many teens need extra help. You are doing the right thing by asking for help. It could save your teen's life.

When should I get help?

- Your teen feels like a stranger to you. You can't talk with your teen.
- Your teen looks sick.
- Your teen spends a lot of time alone. He or she does not have any friends.
- Your teen is mean to animals.
- Your teen is always in a bad mood.
- Your teen is getting into trouble with the law.
- You think your teen is taking drugs or doing other unsafe things.
- Your teen is failing at school.
- Your teen is losing a lot of weight.
- Your teen complains of aches and pains.
- Your teen seems tired all the time.
- Your teen does not want to do anything.
- You are worried about your teen.

Read this book for a full list of other times to get help.

Teen Issues

3

Notes

_____

_____

_____

_____

_____

_____

_____

_____

_____

_____

_____

_____

_____

Friends

What is it?

Friends are teens that like each other. They spend a lot of time together.

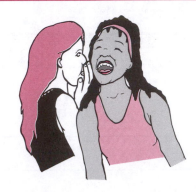

Did you know?

- Friends around the same age are called peers.

- Teens need friends. Friends help teens learn and grow.

- A teen's friends can be more important than family. Teens may want to spend more time with friends than with family.

- There are two kinds of friends; "good" friends and "bad" friends. Good friends help teens to be their best. They help teens build high self-esteem. Bad friends make teens do things that are wrong.

- Teens want to fit in with their friends. That is why it is important for teens to choose the right friends. Teens want to:
    - Dress the way their friends dress.
    - Eat what their friends eat.
    - Act the way their friends act.
    - Do what their friends do.

Friends

- Girls often have one best friend. They spend hours talking. They share their feelings.

- Boys often hang out with several friends. They do things together.

- Teens often do what their friends tell them. This is called peer pressure. Teens don't want to be different. They don't want to lose their friends.

- Peer pressure can make teens do good things like:

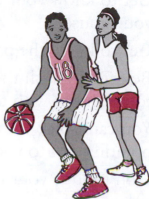

  - Study and get good grades.

  - Join a club.

  - Do sports.

  - Get a part-time job.

- Peer pressure can be bad. It can make teens do things that are wrong like:

  - Drink and drive.

  - Drop out of school.

  - Have sex before the teen is ready.

  - Lie and steal.

  - Take drugs.

- Teens who are close to their family don't give in as often to bad peer pressure.

What can I do?

- Talk with your teen every day. Be part of your teen's life. Show that you care. Know what your teen is doing.

Friends

- Help your teen find good friends. A church group or school club is a place to find good friends. Some good groups for teens are:
  - The YMCA
  - Candy Stripers at hospitals
  - Girl Scouts and Boy Scouts of America
- Get to know your teen's friends. Invite them to your house.
- Get to know the parents of your teen's friends.
- Be friendly with the friends you like. Invite them to do things with the family.
- You can't pick your teen's friends. You can help by pointing out to your teen things you see.
- Don't judge your teen's friends by how they look.
- Talk to your teen at an early age about friends. Teach your teen that good friends are those who:
  - Support you.
  - Care about you.
  - Are fun to be with.
  - Make you feel good about yourself.
- Teach your teen that bad friends are those who:
  - Try to control you.
  - Put you down.
  - Get mad at you all the time.
  - Pressure you to do things.
  - Hurt your feelings.
  - Make you feel that you are not good enough.

- Talk with your teen about peer pressure. Practice with your teen what to say or do when friends try to make your teen do something wrong. This is called role-playing. You can play the friend and your teen can be himself.

- It hurts to lose a friend. Comfort your teen if he or she loses a friend.

- Your teen may want to spend all his time with friends. Find ways to stay close to your teen (see family time on page 19).

When should I get help?

- Your teen does not have any friends.
- Your teen is very shy.
- You think your teen is with the wrong friends.
- Your teen will not let you meet his or her friends.

School

What is it?

School prepares teens for life. It teaches them the skills they need.

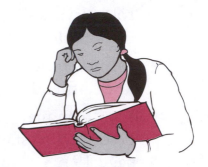

Did you know?

- Teens do better in school if their parents are involved.

- Some teens do poorly in school. There are reasons why this happens.

    - Some teens don't know how to study. They don't know how to take notes in class. They don't know how to use the library.

    - Some teens have problems learning. This is called a learning disability.

    - Some teens are lazy. They don't like to do homework. They don't try.

- Learning disabilities often run in families. Here are some signs of a learning disability:

    - Mixing up letters or numbers. Teen may write 89 instead of 98 or "left" instead of "felt."

    - Having a hard time reading out loud.

    - Having trouble writing papers.

    - Handwriting that is hard to read.

    - Trouble remembering facts.

- Homework can be hard for teens. Some teens stay up late doing homework. They feel a lot of stress.

- Some parents put too much pressure on their teen to do well in school. This can cause stress, depression, or other problems.

- Computers are a tool to help teens do well in school. It is also a good place to find local movies and other things. Teens need to know how to stay safe when using the computer.

What can I do?

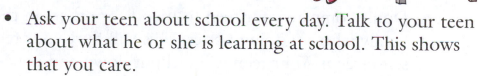

- Show your teen that you care about learning. Go to the library. Take classes.

- Reading gets easier the more you do it. Good reading skills make school easier. Read books in front of your teen. Teach your teen to read for fun.

- Ask your teen about school every day. Talk to your teen about what he or she is learning at school. This shows that you care.

- Show your teen that school is important. Be part of your teen's school. Go to open house and all school meetings. Meet your teen's teachers. Do this even if your teen is doing well at school.

- Know the rules at your teen's school. Talk with your teen about the rules. For example, what happens if a teen is caught smoking? What about drugs? What if a teen brings a knife to school?

- Know how your teen is doing in school. Look over your teen's schoolwork. Ask questions. Praise your teen.

- If your teen is not doing well at school, find out why. Meet with your teen's teachers.

- There are many reasons why your teen may not be doing well:

  - Your teen may need help to plan his time.

  - Your teen may be too busy.

  - Your teen may have a learning disability.

  - Your teen may need some extra help with schoolwork.

- Watch for signs that your teen studies all the time. Help your teen balance school work and fun.

- Don't make your teen study things you like. Support your teen's own interests. Help your teen find what he or she is good at.

- Don't compare your teen to friends or others in the family who are doing better. This will hurt your teen's self-esteem. Your teen will feel put down and may stop trying at school.

- Don't put too much pressure on your teen. Not all teens can get straight A's. If your teen is working hard and gets B's or C's, that's good.

- Praise your teen's hard work and effort. Say things like "I can see you worked hard on this paper. I'm proud of you." This will build your teen's self-esteem.

- Don't get angry if your teen fails a test or class. Stay calm. Try to find out why your teen failed. Never say things like "You're stupid" or "You're lazy." This will hurt your teen's feelings and self-esteem.

- Special teachers can help your teen. They are called tutors. Get a tutor if your teen is getting poor grades.

- Don't do your teen's homework. Your teen must do his or her own homework. There are some ways you can help:

  - Make sure your teen has a quiet, well-lit place to do homework.

  - Talk to your teen about school projects. Help your teen come up with good ideas.

  - Set limits on TV time and video games.

  - Sit nearby and read a book.

  - Bring your teen a snack.

  - Make sure your teen gets enough rest.

- Watch for signs that your teen is having problems at school. Some things are:

  - Your teen does not want to go to school.

  - Your teen is often sick and misses school.

  - Your teen says the teacher does not like him.

  - Your teen is caught cheating.

- Get to know your teen's teachers and school counselor. Talk with them about how your teen is doing.

- If you have a computer at home, keep it in the family area. Watch what your teen does on the computer.

- Teach your teen about safe use of the computer.
  - Tell your teen never to trust anyone they meet in a chat room. The person may not be who they say they are. There are adults in chat rooms who say they are teens. They want to meet teens and may harm them.
  - Tell your teen never to agree to meet anyone they met on the Internet. Have your teen tell you if someone asks to meet them.
  - Teens should never give out their real name, address, phone number, their school name, password or their social security number. Have your teen tell you if someone asks them these questions.
  - Have your teen tell you if they get scared by something said in a chat room or in an e-mail.

When should I get help?

- Your teen fails a class.
- Your teen's grades dropped.
- Your teen is getting into trouble at school.
- You are worried about your teen.
- You and your teen always fight about homework.
- Your teen wants to drop out of school.
- Your teen stopped going to school.
- Your teen has signs of a learning disability (see page 42).
- Tell the police if a person your teen met on the Internet wants to meet your teen.

Exercise

What is it?

Body movement that makes the heart and breathing go faster.

Did you know?

- Regular exercise builds strong bodies. Exercise is also good for other reasons:
  - It helps with stress.
  - It can be fun.
  - It controls appetite and weight.
  - It can help you feel better.
  - It helps you think more clearly.
- Many teens don't get enough exercise. They watch too much TV. Some teens watch 20–25 hours of TV a week. Teens also spend a lot of time on the phone, on the Internet, or playing video games.
- There are many things a teen can do for exercise such as:
  - Bike riding
  - Dancing
  - Jogging
  - Walking the dog
  - Swimming
  - Sports

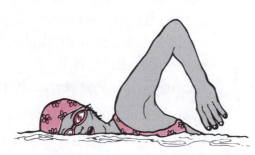

- Some teens exercise too much and become too thin. This is a sign of other problems (see page 55).

- Girls can stop having periods from too much exercise.

- Teens can get hurt from exercising the wrong way.

What can I do?

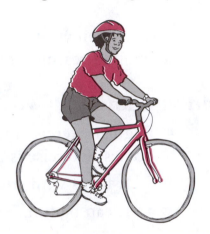

- Help your teen to be active. Limit time watching TV, playing video games, and sitting around.

- Help your teen set exercise goals. Praise your teen for being active.

- Tell your teen how good he or she looks from exercise.

- Exercise with your teen. Go on runs or walks together. It's a good time to talk with your teen.

- Help your teen be safe during exercise. Make sure your teen wears the right shoes. Teens need to wear a helmet for biking, skateboarding, riding scooters, and other activities.

- Watch for signs that your teen is exercising too much. Some signs are losing weight and sore muscles.

Exercise

- Teach your teen to do these things if he or she hurts or pulls a muscle. Use the word RICE to remember what to do:

  - **R**est the area that hurts.
  - **I**ce the area for 30 minutes every 4 hours for 24 hours.
  - **C**ompress or wrap the area.
  - **E**levate (raise) the hurt area higher than the heart.

- Teens learn by example. Get the whole family to exercise. Go for a fast walk in the evening. Go biking on weekends. Exercise is a good way for the family to spend time together.

When should I get help?

- Your teen refuses to be active and is putting on weight.
- Your teen exercises too much and is losing too much weight.
- Your teen has pain or swelling that does not get better with care at home.

Sports

What is it?

It is a game with rules and physical activity.

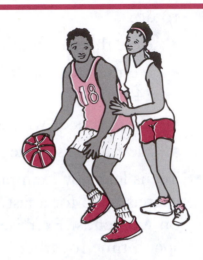

Did you know?

- Sports are good for teens for many reasons.

    - It's good exercise.

    - It keeps teens busy and out of trouble.

    - It teaches teens how to work as part of a team.

    - It's a way to make friends.

    - Sports build skills and self-esteem.

    - It teaches teens how to be good winners and losers.

- Girls who are in sports have better self-esteem and less depression.

- Some teens get hurt doing sports. They may break bones, lose teeth, or pull muscles. Some injuries can last for a lifetime.

- Some coaches and parents work teens too hard. They put too much pressure on teens to win. This can be bad for teens.

- Sports should be fun for teens. It should be something to look forward to.

- Some teens take drugs to play better sports. The drug is called steroids. It makes them stronger and bigger. These drugs are bad for many reasons:

  - Taking steroids is bad for the heart and liver.

  - Steroids can make boys sterile (unable to father a baby).

  - They give girls body hair and make the breasts smaller. These changes don't go away when the teen stops taking steroids.

- Teens need some free time. Some teens do too many sports. They are too busy. They don't have time to sleep or study. They are always rushed and stressed.

What can I do?

- Let your teen choose a sport. Don't push your teen to follow your dreams.

- Support your teen. Go to games. Let your teen know you think sports are good. Tell your teen you are proud of him or her.

- Don't stress winning. Stress playing fair and having fun.

- Teach your teen to be a good winner and loser. Watch how you act at your teen's games.

  - Don't lose control.

  - Don't use bad language.

- - Don't get angry.
  - Don't argue with the referee or coach.

- Praise your teen after a game, even if the team lost. Talk about how hard everyone worked. Talk about good plays that were made. Your teen will learn that what is important is how a person plays the game.

- After a game, don't tell your teen things he or she did wrong. This will make your teen feel bad. Tell your teen how proud you are.

- Keep your teen safe. Make sure your teen wears the right shoes, pads, and other safety wear. Make sure it is in good condition.

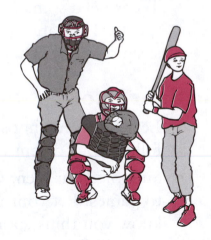

- Teach your teen to listen to his or her body. Pain means something is wrong. Your teen needs to stop if something pops, hurts, or doesn't feel right.

- Teach your teen what to do if he or she hurts or pulls a muscle. Use the word RICE to remember what to do:
  - **R**est the area that hurts.
  - **I**ce the area for 30 minutes every 4 hours for 24 hours.
  - **C**ompress or wrap the area.
  - **E**levate (raise) the injured area higher than the heart.

- Watch for signs that your teen is being pushed too hard. Some things are:
  - Your teen plays sports when hurt or in pain.
  - Your teen is on a special diet that does not seem right to you.
  - Your teen's school grades drop.
  - Sports take up all your teen's time. There is little time to study or go out.
  - Your teen is losing or gaining a lot of weight.
- Don't let your teen play sports when he or she is sick. A sick teen can get hurt.
- Tell your teen to never take drugs to get bigger or stronger. These drugs will hurt his or her body for life. Watch for signs that your teen may be taking drugs to get stronger.
- Teens in sports need to eat the right foods. Keep lots of healthy food in the house. Help your teen pack snacks for school.

When should I get help?

- Your teen has bad pain.
- Your teen has pain or swelling that does not go away in a few days.
- Your teen is not eating right.
- Your teen is gaining or losing a lot of weight.
- Your teen is failing at school.
- Sports are the only thing your teen wants to do.

Eating Problems

What is it?

It's an unhealthy way of eating that a teen cannot stop.
There are three eating problems that teens can have.
They are called eating disorders.

- Eating very little food and becoming too thin.
  This is called anorexia.

- Eating large amounts of food. Teen then gets rid
  of the food by throwing up or taking laxatives
  (over-the-counter medicine). This is called bulimia.

- Eating too much food and gaining a lot of weight.
  This is called compulsive overeating.

Did you know?

- Most teens with eating problems are girls.

- Most teens with eating problems need help from an
  outside expert. Without help, a teen can die.

- Teens with eating problems often have few friends.
  They spend a lot of time alone. They worry about food
  and how they look.

- Many teens want to look like the movie stars they see.
  This can cause eating problems.

Teen eats too little (anorexia):

- Anorexia is a very serious illness. It starts as a diet to
  lose a few pounds. Once the weight is lost, the teen
  can't stop dieting.

Eating Problems

- Anorexia often starts when a teen is young. It can go on for many years.

- Teens with this problem eat very little. They starve themselves to be thin. They often exercise a lot to get even thinner.

- A teen with this problem looks very sick. Here are some signs:
  - Teen is very thin, just skin and bones.
  - Teen has dry skin and thin hair.
  - Monthly periods stop.
  - Teen feels cold all the time.
  - Fine hairs grow on the arms, back, and face.
  - Teen is weak and depressed.

- Even though the teen is very thin, she thinks she's fat. She is afraid of gaining weight.

- A teen with anorexia loses her body curves. She looks like a child again.

- Her self-esteem is tied to how thin she is. The only thing that matters is being thin.

- A teen with anorexia denies she has a problem. She is very sick. She can die without help.

Teen eats large amounts of food and throws up or takes laxatives after eating (bulimia):

- Bulimia often starts in the later teen years.

- Teens with this problem eat a lot of food in a short time. This is called binge eating. They binge alone or with friends.

- Binge eating often happens when a teen feels stress. Teens also do it when they are lonely or upset.

- They eat high-calorie "junk" food like ice cream and cookies.

- They feel guilty after the binge. They make themselves throw up right after eating. They do this so they won't get fat. Many teens also take laxatives to get the food out of their body.

- It can be hard to tell that a teen has bulimia. The teen's weight often stays the same. Here are some signs to watch for:
  - Trips to the bathroom right after meals.
  - Large amounts of food missing from the house.
  - Tooth decay from throwing up often.
  - Puffy face near the ears.
  - Cuts and dry skin on the hands and fingers.
  - Mood swings.
  - Muscle cramps.
  - Burning in the chest.
  - Feeling tired.

- Teens with bulimia know they have a problem. They try to keep it a secret.

- Bulimia is a serious problem. A teen can die without help.

Teen eats too much food and gets fat (compulsive overeating):

- Teens with this eating problem can't limit how much food they eat.

- They use food to feel better.
- The overeating often starts as a child.
- Problems with weight often run in families. Overweight parents tend to have fat children.
- Sometimes overeating in a teen can start with a crisis like an accident. The teen eats too much and gets fat. The overeating does not stop after the crisis is over.

What can I do?

- Eat healthy and exercise. Teach your teen to do the same.
- Serve healthy foods in the right amounts. The website **www.mypyramid.gov** can tell you what food your teen needs to eat.
- Teens need to eat three meals and two snacks a day. They need to eat food every day from each of the five food groups.
  - Bread (whole grain), cereal, rice, and pasta
  - Vegetables
  - Fruits
  - Meat, fish, poultry, eggs, and nuts
  - Milk, yogurt, and cheese (low fat or nonfat)
- Give your teen foods high in iron. Teens need to eat foods rich in iron because they are growing. Girls need extra iron due to their monthly periods. Some foods high in iron are:
  - Meats
  - Spinach
  - Raisins
  - Beans
  - Cereals and breads with added iron

- Try to eat meals together as a family.

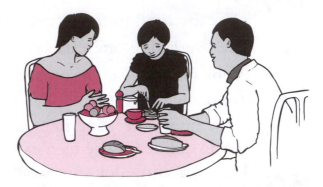

- Teach your teen healthy eating habits.

Don't do these things:

- Don't make your teen eat all the food on his or her plate. Your teen should stop eating when full.

- Don't use food as a reward. For example, don't give extra cake for doing well on a test.

- Don't use food to make your teen feel better. When your teen is sad, talk with your teen. Eating doesn't help.

- Don't use food to punish your teen.

- Watch for signs that your teen may have an eating problem.

- Don't talk about dieting around your teen.

- Notice if your teen goes to the bathroom right after meals.

- Take your teen to the doctor if you are worried. Don't believe your teen when she says she is OK.

When should I get help?

- Your teen has gained or lost a lot of weight.
- Your teen refuses many meals.
- Your teen is always on a diet and is afraid to gain weight.
- Your teen exercises too much.
- Your teen looks sick.
- Your teen has some signs of an eating problem.
- Your teen is thin but says "I'm fat."
- Your teen takes laxatives to go to the bathroom.

Anger

What is it?

Anger is a strong feeling that makes a person ready to fight.

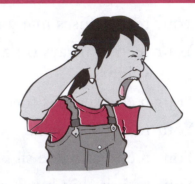

Did you know?

- Anger is a normal feeling. But it is not normal to be angry all the time.

- Many teens get angry often. Some teens have trouble controlling their anger. Anger that is not controlled can lead to harm.

- Teens get angry with their parents for many reasons.

- It's not easy to stay calm when a person is angry.

- Teens learn by example. They deal with anger the way adults do. Parents need to control their anger.

- Yelling does not help. Things said in anger can hurt a person.

- Anger can cover up depression.

What can I do?

- Watch for signs that your teen is angry. Talk with your teen about why he or she is angry. Help your teen find the real reason for the anger. Your teen may feel better knowing what is wrong.

Anger

- Your teen will often get angry with you. Don't give in just because your teen is angry. If you do, you will teach your teen that anger gets them what they want. It is OK to give in if you are wrong.

- Teach your teen to feel the signs that he or she is getting angry. Knowing the signs can help control anger. Some things to notice are:
    - Fast heartbeat and breathing.
    - Feeling in a bad mood.
    - Flushed cheeks.
    - Butterflies in the stomach.
    - Tight muscles in the throat and chest.
    - Urge to hurt someone.

- Teach your teen ways to deal with anger. The best way is to find the problem causing the anger and fix it.

- Sometimes your teen doesn't know why he is angry. Your teen may know the problem but can't fix it. Teach your teen healthy ways to deal with anger such as:
    - Talk about feelings with a friend.
    - Go for a walk or jog.
    - Work out in a gym.
    - Paint or draw.
    - Write about feelings.
    - Punch a bag or pillow.
    - Count backwards or take deep breaths.

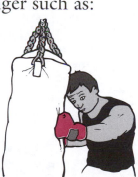

- Teach your teen by example how to control anger and how to forgive.

Anger

When should I get help?

- Your teen always seems angry.
- Your teen gets violent when angry.
- Your teen cannot control his anger.
- You are afraid your teen may hurt himself or someone else.
- You cannot control your anger.
- You are always angry at your teen.

Violence

What is it?

Violence is doing harm to people or things. Bullying is a form of violence.

Did you know?

- Teens see violence all around them. It's in the movies, on TV, and in the news. Many video games are very violent.

- Violence in school often starts with kids making fun of others. This is called bullying. It is a serious problem.

- Bullying is when a teen is picked on over and over by another teen or group of teens. Bullies pick on teens they think do not fit in. Bullies attack by name calling, hitting, kicking and tripping a teen. Bullies may send nasty e-mails to a teen.

- Bullies need to be stopped. If they are not stopped, they can become more violent.

- Most bullies are big boys. Many bullies are unhappy. They do poorly in school. They have problems at home. They have low self-esteem.

- Teens who are bullied are small, quiet, and weak. They have low self-esteem. They have few friends. They are easy targets for bullies.

- Teens who are bullied get anxious and afraid. They are at risk for health problems, depression and suicide. Teens who are bullied need help.

- Some teens may get violent and want to use a gun if they can get one.

- Parents are responsible if a teen uses their gun. This is true even if the gun is kept locked.

What can I do?

- Teach your teen that violence is wrong. It is not the way to solve problems. Talk about non-violent ways to solve problems.

- Be non-violent at home. Don't take your anger out on people, pets, or things. Teach your teen healthy ways to deal with anger (see page 61).

- Talk about what happens to people who are violent. The "bad" guys don't get away with violence in real life. Talk about people in the news who were violent and got caught.

- Listen to the words in the music your teen listens to. Talk about bad or violent words and why they are wrong.

- Help your teen stay safe. Talk about places, people, and things to avoid. Here are some things to tell your teen:

  - Stay away from dark parking lots.

  - Don't use public rest rooms alone.

  - Plan safe places to go.

  - Always know where the local police station is located.

Violence

- Tell your teen that being a bully is wrong. Talk with your teen about what to do if he or she sees someone being a bully:
    - Never join in. It is wrong.
    - Report bullying to a teacher, coach or school counselor.
- Your teen may not tell you that he or she is being bullied. Watch for these signs:
    - Your teen is afraid to go out.
    - Your teen does not want to go to school.
    - Your teen has signs of body harm or torn clothes.
    - School grades drop.
- If your teen is being bullied at school, get help right away.
    - Meet with the school principal.
    - Make a plan to stop it.
    - Tell your teen what to do, like walk away and get help from an adult.
- Look for signs that a teen is at risk of being violent:
    - Teen bullies others.
    - Teen is bullied by others.
    - Teen has few friends.
    - Teen makes violent threats when angry.
    - Teen is mean to animals.
    - Teen watches violent movies.
    - Teen plays violent video games.

Violence

- Teen writes about anger and violence.
- Teen is often sad or has mood swings.

- Guns in the home are a big risk. The best thing to do is to get rid of the gun. If you don't want to get rid of the gun, do these things:
  - Tell your teen that he or she is not allowed to touch the gun.
  - Keep the gun locked up at all times.
  - Store bullets separate from the gun.
  - Talk with your teen about the danger of guns.

When should I get help?
- Your teen can't control his or her temper.
- Your teen is violent.
- You are afraid your teen might hurt someone.
- Your teen has been the victim of violence.
- Your teen is a bully.
- Your teen is being picked on by others.
- You are afraid your teen might hurt him or herself.

Depression

What is it?

It is feeling sad, down, or blue for longer than a few hours or a day. The feeling is so strong it changes how a teen looks and acts.

Did you know?

- Most teens feel sad or feel down at times. The feeling usually passes in a few hours or a day.

- 1 in 5 teens are depressed.

- Twice as many girls as boys feel depressed at times. Girls get depressed about their body and how they look.

- Teens may get depressed about what their peers say about them on the Internet.

- Teens often say, "I'm depressed" or "I'm sad." This happens for many reasons. If the mood or feeling passes in a few hours or a day, it's normal.

- Sometimes the sad feelings don't go away. They get deeper and go on for days and weeks. The teen may start to feel that things will never get better. This is called feeling hopeless. Teens who have real depression start to look and act different.

- Signs of depression are:
  - Less interest in school or friends.
  - School grades drop.

- Less interest in things teen used to like.
- Teen is angry or mean.
- Change in appetite (eating too much or too little).
- Change in sleep (sleeping too much or too little).
- Low energy, always tired.
- Teen does not wash or dress like before.
- Spends a lot of time alone.
- Complains of pains or other health problems.

- Teens who are depressed need outside help. Some teens need to take medicine or go to a hospital.

- If a teen does not get help, he or she may try to harm him or herself.

What can I do?

- Talk with your teen when he or she is feeling sad or is upset. Talking about feelings can help your teen feel better. Sit down and show that you care.

- Help your teen to share feelings by saying things like:
  - I can see that you are hurting.
  - Tell me how you are feeling.
  - Tell me more.

- Show your teen that his or her feelings are important. Think back to when you were a teen and how you felt.

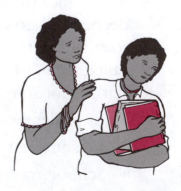

- Tell your teen that you love him or her and that you are there to help.

Depression

- Tell your teen you want to understand how he or she is feeling.

- Don't make fun of what your teen tells you. It may seem like a little thing to you but it's a big problem to your teen.

- Don't get angry about what your teen says. Just listen. Control your feelings.

- Tell your teen that it is OK to feel sad sometimes. These sad feelings will go away. Talk about things your teen can do to feel better. Things like exercise can help.

- Help your teen learn what to do when things go wrong. Help your teen learn how to solve problems.

- Watch for signs of depression (see list on pages 67–68).

When should I get help?

- Your teen is sad or depressed often.

- You are not sure if your teen's mood swings are normal.

- Your teen's appetite, sleep, or energy has changed.

- Your teen is giving things away.

- Your teen has lost interest in doing things. He or she spends a lot of time alone, cries a lot, or is angry and mean.

- Your teen has trouble studying. He or she is failing at school.

- Your teen started getting into trouble, using drugs or alcohol, or doing other bad things.

- You are worried about your teen.

Suicide

What is it?

Suicide is killing oneself.

Did you know?

- Each year 8 out of 100 teens **try** to kill themselves.
- Suicide is the third leading cause of death among teens.
- Girls try suicide more often. Boys succeed in killing themselves more often.
- Some teens try suicide more than once.
- Beware of a sudden change in a teen's mood. It could mean that a teen has decided to take his or her life.
- Some things can put a troubled teen at greater risk for suicide such as:
  - Divorce.
  - Death of a close family member or friend.
  - Death of a pet.
  - Failing at school.
  - Breakup with a boyfriend or girlfriend.
  - Using drugs or alcohol.
  - Getting pregnant.

Suicide

- There are places to call to get help right away. They are called suicide hotlines. You can find the phone number in the phone book or call 411.

- Some teens need to be put in a hospital to keep them safe.

What can I do?

- Watch for signs that your teen may be at risk for suicide. Some signs are:

  - Sadness that does not go away.

  - Anger without a clear reason.

  - Teen feels lost or alone.

  - Loss of interest in friends, activities, and school.

  - Teen starts to give his or her things away.

  - Teen thinks there is no way out.

  - Teen uses drugs or alcohol to feel better.

  - Teen says things like "I should kill myself," or "nothing matters anymore."

  - Teen listens to music about death or suicide.

- Tell your teen every day that he or she is special. Tell your teen that you love him or her very much.

- Tell your teen to come to you for help no matter what he or she did. Everyone makes mistakes. You are there to help.

- When your child comes for help, don't start yelling. Teach your teen how to fix mistakes.

- Teach your teen that life is worth living. Help your teen:
  - See the beauty in the world.
  - See a good future.
  - Find an interest.
  - Find ways to be happy.

- **If your teen talks about suicide, get help right away! Believe what your teen says. Don't think that suicide can't happen in your family. Speak with your doctor about your concerns. Call the National Suicide Prevention line at 1-800-273-8255 for help.**

- Don't put too much pressure on your teen. Don't make your teen feel like he or she can never please you.

- Spend time listening and talking with your teen. Help your teen find hope. Let your teen know there are things that can be done.

- Read your teen's diary if it is left out. It may be your teen's way of asking for help. Do this **only** if you are worried about your teen's safety.

- If you think your teen is at risk for suicide, call your doctor right away. Your teen may need medicine. Your teen may need to go to a hospital.

- Spend more time with your teen. Be there when your teen comes home from school. Remove guns, kitchen knives, and all medicines (including over-the-counter medicines) from your house.

- Never give up on your teen.

Suicide

When should I get help?

- Your teen talks about death or suicide or says things like "I wish I were dead."

- Your teen writes about death.

- Your teen gives things away.

- Your teen seems depressed and does not want to do anything.

- You are worried about your teen.

- You think your teen is at risk for suicide.

- If your teen tries to hurt him or herself, get help right away.

Dating and Sex

4

Dating

What is it?

Dating is going out with
someone a person likes.
Dating can be two teens
going out or a group of teens.

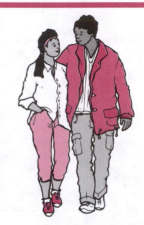

Did you know?

- Parents have rules for dating. Age 16 is a common
  age for parents to let a teen date. Some teens want to
  date at 12 or 13.

- Each teen is different. Teens are not ready for dating
  at the same age. Dating rules need to be set for each
  teen. Just because a sister or brother started dating at
  one age doesn't mean the next child has to start at the
  same age.

- Dating can mean
  driving in a car
  with another
  person. Read
  about driving on
  page 124.

- Group dating
  means couples going out together.
  This is very common.

- Early, steady dating often leads to sex.

Dating

- Curfew is the time a teen needs to be at home. A curfew is good because:
  - It keeps teens from staying out too late, when they could get into trouble.
  - It gives teens the duty to be home by a special time.
  - It gives parents peace of mind knowing what time their teen will be home.

What can I do?

- Encourage group dating as often as possible.
- Don't let your teen date older people (no more than one year older).
- Help your teen think of fun things to do on a date.
- Talk with your teen about who will pay for the date. It may be a good idea to have both teens share in the cost.
- Discuss how to say "no" to sex before your teen starts dating. Read about sex on page 84.
- If your teen starts to date before he drives, offer to be the driver.
- Meet your teen's date or at least know the date's name and phone number.
- Make sure your teen has money to call you or to take a bus or taxi home.
- Tell your teen what time he or she needs to be home. Make it early at first. You can make it later as your teen gets older, or for special dates like a school dance.

- Tell your teen to call you if he or she is going to get home late.

- Try to be there when your teen comes home from a date. Talk with your teen about how things went. Don't be too pushy.

- If your teen is dating someone you don't like, talk with your teen about it. Tell your teen your concerns about the other person.

- Talk with your teen about good things to look for in other teens.

When should I get help?

- Your teen is dating a person you think will get him or her into trouble. You tried talking with your teen but he or she won't stop dating this person.

Date Rape

What is it?

Date rape is when one person on a date forces the other person to have sex. It's also rape if a person has sex with someone who is too drunk or high on drugs to know what is happening.

Did you know?

- Rape is a crime. A person who rapes someone can go to jail.

- It is never OK to rape someone. People don't "ask" to be raped by the clothes they wear or the way they act.

- If a person says no to sex, the other person should stop. Teens need to be taught that **no** means **no**.

- A person can say no at any time. Heavy kissing and touching doesn't mean a teen wants to have sex.

- Some teens may think they should get sex in return for paying for a date. This is not true. A girl and boy should talk before a date about who will pay. Sex is not a pay back.

- There are drugs that can be put in a person's drink. A person who takes the drug can be raped without knowing it. These drugs are called date rape drugs.

- A person who is raped needs help from a doctor, nurse, or social worker. The person must not shower before they see a doctor.

- There are rape crisis centers to help people who have been raped. You can find the phone number in the phone book or call 411.

What can I do?

- Talk with your teen about date rape.
- To avoid date rape, teach your teen these things:
  - Have first dates in a group if possible or in a public place.
  - Make sure no one puts anything in your drink.
  - Don't get drunk or take drugs.
  - Don't let your date get drunk or take drugs.
  - Stay with other people at parties. Don't go off alone with your date.
  - Bring money so you can call home or take a bus or taxi.
  - Stop before kissing gets too hot.
  - Talk to your date about sex. Agree that if one person says no, it means no.
- Boys and girls can be charged with statutory rape and go to jail if they have sex with someone under the legal age (16 or 18 depending on the state). This can happen even if the person under age agrees to have sex.

When should I get help?

- If a teen is raped, take the teen to a hospital right away. Tell them it is not their fault. Tell them not to shower or wash before going to the hospital.

Not Having Sex (Abstinence)

What is it?

Abstinence means not having sex.

Did you know?

- Not having sex is 100% safe in preventing pregnancy. It is almost 100% safe in preventing sexually transmitted diseases (STDs).

- It may be hard for a teen not to have sex.

    - Friends may say they are having sex. But this may not be true.

    - Teens may feel they are in love. They may want to have sex because of these feelings.

    - Teens see sex on TV and in the movies.

- Teens need a lot of support not to have sex. They need people to say its OK not to have sex.

- Not having sex keeps a teen:

    - Free from worry about getting pregnant.

    - Free from sexually transmitted diseases (STDs).

    - Free from loss of self-respect.

    - Free to have lots of friends of both sexes.

    - Able to focus on sports, work, and school.

Not Having Sex (Abstinence)

- Teens who had sex can decide not to have sex again.

- Many churches, temples, and other places have support groups for teens who don't want to have sex.

- Sex does not make a teen part of an "in" group. It does not help a teen keep friends or stop feeling lonely.

- There are many ways teens can show they care:

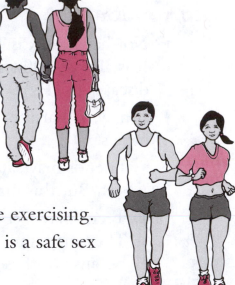

  - Hugs and kisses.

  - Holding hands.

  - Talking about feelings.

  - Writing love poems or letters.

  - Buying each other gifts.

  - Talking on the phone.

  - Doing things together like exercising.

- Masturbation (see page 115) is a safe sex activity.

What can I do?

- Talk with your teen about not having sex. Tell your teen that not having sex is OK.

- Teach your teen about condoms and birth control. Teens who don't plan to have sex still need to know about these things.

- Talk with your teen about how he or she feels about sex. Plan what you will say if your teen asks you what you did as a teen. Share what you learned from your actions.

Not Having Sex (Abstinence)

- Talk about other things your teen can do to show he or she cares.
- Help your teen find a support group.
- Talk with your teen about how to say NO to sex. Here are some things your teen can say:
  - "I'm not ready to have sex."
  - "Please respect my choice not to have sex."
  - "If you are only going out with me to have sex, lets stop now."
  - "If you love me, you wouldn't want me to do something I'm not ready for."
  - "I don't care if everybody is doing it. I'm not ready."
  - "Even though I had sex with you before, I made a mistake. I don't want to have sex again."
- Spend time with your teen. Do things together. Show your teen that there are lots of fun things to do.
- Don't accuse your teen of having sex because of something you heard.

When should I get help?

- Call your local church, temple, or YMCA and ask about groups and activities that support teens not to have sex.
- Call these groups for information:
  - True Love Waits, 1-800-588-9248
  - The National Abstinence Clearinghouse, 1-888-577-2966

Sex

What is it?

Sex is the act of putting the penis into the vagina. This is also called intercourse. Oral sex is when the penis is put into the mouth or the mouth is put over a girl's genitals. If the penis is put in the anus, it is called anal sex. Other words for sex are getting laid, going all the way, doing it, going to bed, making love, sleeping with someone. Coitus and copulation also mean sex.

Did you know?

- Children see sex on TV and in the movies. It's in music, books, and other places.

- Children need to learn the facts about sex.

- It's good to begin talking to children about sex at the age of 8 or 9, before their bodies start to change.

- Teens need to know about sex, birth control, and sexually transmitted diseases (STDs) before they start to date or have sex.

- Talking about sex does not make teens want to have sex.

- Most schools have sex education classes that teach the facts about sex. Parents teach children about values.

- Teens often learn about sex from their friends. What they learn may not be right.

Sex

- Many teens have sex before they are ready. This happens because:
  - They don't know how to say **No** to sex.
  - They are afraid of being different.
  - Their friends talk them into having sex. This is called peer pressure.
  - They want to please their date.
- Many teens who had sex wish they had not.
- Here are some questions for teens who are thinking about having sex:
  - Do you feel different because you never had sex?
  - Do you know how to protect yourself from pregnancy and STDs?
  - Are you being pressured into having sex?
  - Will having sex change how you feel about yourself?
- Just because a teen had sex does not mean he or she has to have sex again. A teen can decide anytime not to have sex.

What can I do?

- Read and learn about sex yourself.
- Be open and honest with your child about sex from a young age. Always answer your child's questions. Make it OK for your child to ask questions.
- Don't lecture about sex.

- Use the right words for the genital parts.

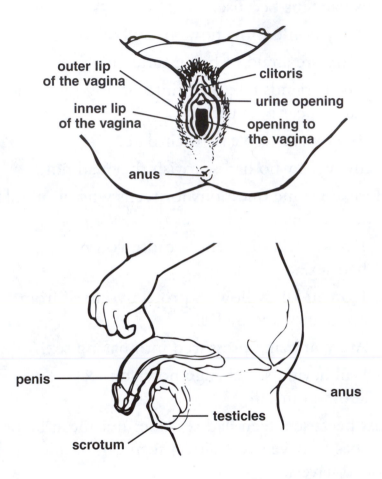

- Start talking with your teen about sex by asking questions like:
  - What are you learning in school about sex?
  - What are your friends saying about sex?
  - What do you know about STDs?
- There are many groups that you and your teen can attend to learn about sex. Your church may have a teen

and parent group. The YMCA or the local boys and girls club may have groups.

- Help your teen plan what to say if he or she is being pressured into having sex:
  - Stop I want to go home now!
  - I'm not ready to have sex.
  - Don't pressure me to have sex with you. I don't want to.
  - I don't need to prove my love by having sex.
  - If you love me, you will wait.
- Tell your teen:
  - It's normal to dream about sex.
  - It's OK to talk about sex.
  - You don't have to have sex to fit in or be cool.

When should I get help?

- You don't understand some things about sex.
- You don't feel comfortable talking with your teen about sex.
- Your teen is having sex. You want birth control for your teen.
- You want your teen checked for STDs or pregnancy. The visit is private between the doctor and your teen. The doctor can't talk to you about the visit unless your teen says it's OK.

Safer Sex

What is it?

Safer sex means using a condom during vaginal, anal, and oral sex. This keeps the man's sperm from going inside the partner. It also keeps body fluids away from each other.

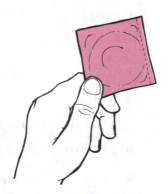

Did you know?

- A condom is sometimes called a rubber, love glove, safe, sheath, Trojan, or balloon.

- A condom should be put on as soon as the penis is hard.

- Condoms help stop the spread of most sexually transmitted diseases (STDs). Condoms work only when used the right way.

- Using a condom every time is each person's duty.

- Many people who have a sexually transmitted disease (STD) don't know it. They don't have any signs. They look and feel well.

- Condoms are not good forever. There is a date on the outside wrap. Check the date before using the condom. If the date has passed, the condom is no longer good. It should be thrown away.

- Here's how to use a condom:

Step 1
Squeeze the center of the condom package to get the air out. If there is no air, the condom is no good. Throw it away.

Step 2
Open the package with care. Be sure not to tear the condom with your nails or teeth.

Step 3
Men with foreskins (uncircumcised) should pull back the foreskin first.

Step 4
Put the condom over the tip of the penis. Make sure the ring of the condom is on the outside.

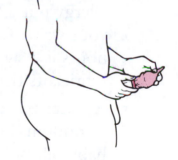

Step 5
Squeeze the air out of the tip of the condom. Hold the tip of the condom with one hand. Unroll the condom to the base of the penis with the other hand.

- If the condom does not unroll, it's on wrong. Throw it away. Start over with a new condom.

- After sex, hold the condom and pull the penis out slowly.

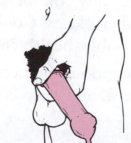

- Slide the condom off. Throw the condom away. Never use the same condom more than one time.

- Don't use two condoms at the same time. It is not as safe as one condom.

- Latex condoms are best. Don't use lambskin condoms. They don't protect against STDs.

- Some people are allergic to latex. Signs of allergy are redness, itching, and burning in the vagina or penis. People who are allergic to latex can use plastic (polyurethane) condoms.

- Some condoms have a spermicide that kills sperm. It is called nonoxynol-9.

- There are creams to put in the vagina that also have nonoxynol-9. They are good to use with a condom.

- Some people are allergic to spermicides. To test for allergy put a little bit of spermicide on the inside of your wrist. Redness or itching in the area after a few hours is a sign of allergy. If allergic, use condoms and lubricants that don't have spermicides.

- A water-based lubricant like K-Y jelly can be used with a condom. Don't use oil-based lubricants like Vaseline, baby oil, or hand lotion with condoms. They can make condoms break.

- You can buy condoms at drugstores, grocery stores, and other places. Condoms cost about $1.00 each. Some public health clinics give condoms away free.

- Keep condoms in a cool, dry place like a purse or shirt pocket. Don't keep condoms in a car or in a wallet.

- Condoms don't stop all diseases. A person can still get lice, scabies, genital warts, or herpes while using a condom.

- A dental dam should be used for oral sex (mouth-to-vagina or mouth-to-anus sex). A dental dam is a thin piece of latex that is put over the vagina or anus. Condoms should be used for mouth-to-penis sex.

What can I do?

- Learn as much as you can about safer sex.

- Teach your teen the right way to use a condom. Have your teen practice putting a condom on a banana.

- Teach your teen that using a condom is each person's duty. Girls can buy condoms as well as boys.

- Go with your teen to buy the first condom. Make sure the condoms are latex and are low cost or free from a clinic.

- There are many types of condoms. Tell your teen to try several types. Your teen will find the one that works best.

- Talk with your teen about safe sex actions like:
  - Kissing with closed lips.
  - Hugging.
  - Rubbing against each other with clothes on.
  - Masturbating alone.

- Teach your teen what to say and do if a partner does not want to use a condom. Teach your teen to always use a condom. Sex without a condom is a big mistake!

- Teach your teen these things about condoms:
  - Condoms protect against pregnancy and STDs.
  - Use a condom each time you have sex.
  - Use a new condom each time.
  - Carry a condom with you.
  - Check the date on the outside wrap. Don't use old condoms.
  - Condoms that are good have air inside the package. Throw the condom away if there is no air.
  - Know how to put a condom on the right way.
  - Put a condom on as soon as the penis is hard.
  - A condom may break.
- Tell your teen what to do if a condom breaks:
  - Stop having sex right away.
  - Take the penis out.
  - The girl needs to go to a family planning clinic within 72 hours (read about emergency contraception on page 107).

When should I get help?

- Your teen may have an STD.
- You are not comfortable talking with your teen about safer sex.
- You can't answer some of your teen's questions.
- You are worried about what your teen is doing.
- Your teen had sex and the condom broke or came off.
- You think your teen may be pregnant.

Sexually Transmitted Diseases (STDs)

What is it?

STDs are diseases or infections spread from one person who has a disease to another person during sexual contact. Sexual contact means vaginal, oral, or anal sex. It also is skin-to-skin contact in the genital areas.

Did you know?

- There are about 25 different STDs.
- About 3 million teens get an STD each year.
- People with STDs often look well. They may not know they have an STD. They can give the STD to a person during sex.
- STDs can be passed during vaginal, anal, or oral sex. You can also get some STDs like genital warts from skin-to-skin contact.
- STDs are spread by body fluids such as blood, vaginal fluids, and semen.
- You can get one or more STDs the first time you have sex with someone who has a disease.
- You can get the same STD many times.
- Some STDs like chlamydia, gonorrhea, and syphilis can be cured.

Sexually Transmitted Diseases (STDs)

- There is no cure for these STDs:
  - HIV/AIDS
  - Genital herpes
  - HPV/Genital warts
  - Hepatitis B

- Here is a list of common STDs:
  - Chlamydia
  - Genital herpes
  - HPV/Genital warts
  - Gonorrhea
  - Hepatitis B
  - HIV/AIDS
  - Trichomonas
  - Crabs
  - Syphilis

- Here are some signs of STDs:
  - Pain or itching in the genitals or sex parts.
  - Fluid (drip or discharge) coming out of the vagina or penis.
  - Burning or itching when peeing (passing urine).
  - Sores, blisters, bumps or rashes on the genitals.
  - Fever, body aches, lower stomach pain.
  - Bad smell from the genitals.

- People must go to the doctor right away if they think they have an STD. Here is what can happen if a person doesn't get medicine for an STD:
  - Boys and girls can get sterile. This means they can never have babies.
  - HPV/Genital warts can cause cancer in women.
  - STDs can cause problems during pregnancy.
  - STDs can be passed to newborn babies.
  - People can die from some STDs.

Sexually Transmitted Diseases (STDs)

- Teens who are sexually active need to always use a condom. They also need to get tested for STDs every 6 months.

- Most clinics will test teens for STDs without a parent's consent.

- There is a vaccine for hepatitis B. All teens need to get this shot (vaccine).

- There is a shot for HPV. It protects against some types of HPV. Girls need to get the shot before they start having sex. The HPV shot prevents cervical cancer.

What can I do?

- Learn as much as you can about STDs.

- Talk with your teen about sex and STDs. Experts say to start when your child is 8 or 9 years old.

- Answer your teen's questions honestly.

- Have your teen read about STDs. Talk with your teen about what he or she read.

- Show your teen pictures of some of the diseases. This will help your teen know why using a condom is so important.

- Support your teen to not have sex.

- Teach your teen how to have safer sex by:

  - Hugging and touching each other with clothes on.

  - Using a condom and cream that contains nonoxynol-9.

  - Using a condom or a dental dam.

- Tell your teen **never** to do these things:
  - Sex without a condom.
  - Oral sex without a condom or dental dam.
  - Share sex toys like vibrators or dildos.
- Some health clinics give away free condoms. Visit one near you to find out about their services.
- Spend time with your teen so you can talk together. Get your teen interested in sports and other things.
- Never tease your teen about sex or STDs. Keep secrets that your teen tells you.
- If your teen is sexually active, tell your teen to get tested for STDs every 6 months.
- If you think your teen has an STD, take him or her to the doctor right away. Make sure your teen tells his or her sex partner about the STD.
- If your teen has an STD, he or she must not have sex until it is cured.
- Make sure your teen gets a shot for hepatitis B.
- Talk to your doctor about the HPV shot. Your teen needs to get the shot before she starts having sex.

When should I get help?

- Your teen is having sex and has signs of an STD (see list on page 94).
- You don't understand STDs. You want someone to talk with your teen.

Sexually Transmitted Diseases (STDs)

- Your teen has an STD. You are worried about your teen.

- You are not comfortable talking with your teen about condoms and STDs.

- To get a shot for HPV and hepatitis B.

HIV/AIDS

What is it?

HIV is a virus that causes AIDS. HIV and AIDS make the body weak and not able to fight disease. People with HIV or AIDS can get sick very easily. First a person gets HIV. Months or years later, HIV causes the disease called AIDS. There is no cure for HIV or AIDS.

Did you know?

- AIDS is a bad disease. People can protect themselves from getting it.
- People get HIV when body fluid with HIV enters their body. This fluid can be blood, semen (the liquid that sperm is in), vaginal fluid, or breast milk.
- HIV is passed from person to person in these ways:
  - Oral, anal, or vaginal sex without a condom with a person who has HIV.
  - Using the same needle or syringe as a person with HIV.
  - An infected mother can pass HIV to her unborn baby.
  - A mother with HIV can pass the virus to her baby by breast-feeding.

- Body piercing and tattooing using tools with the HIV virus on them.

- People with HIV can look healthy for a long time. You can't tell if people have HIV just by looking at them.

- The disease can be passed even when the person has no signs of HIV.

- HIV is not spread by shaking hands, working, playing, or living together. You cannot get HIV from food, water, bugs, or toilet seats.

- Anyone can get HIV and AIDS. Movie stars, doctors, teachers, children, and teens get HIV and AIDS.

- Early signs of HIV can be:

  - Fever
  - Feeling sick
  - Swollen glands
  - Sore throat
  - Diarrhea
  - Rash
  - Feeling tired
  - Joint and muscle pains

- Other diseases can also cause these signs. The only way to be sure is to be tested for HIV.

- A person with HIV can get AIDS in a few months or as long as 10 to 15 years.

- AIDS causes problems like weight loss, diarrhea, and fever. People with AIDS often get bad diseases like T.B., pneumonia, or cancer.

- As soon as a person gets HIV, he or she can pass it to others.

- There are tests that check for HIV and AIDS. A person can get a test at a doctor's office or a health clinic. It takes about 2 weeks to get the results.

- A person can be tested without anyone knowing. Some clinics don't ask for your name.

- There is no cure for HIV and AIDS. There is medicine to slow down the disease. These medicines cost a lot of money. Public health clinics or AIDS organizations can help with the cost.

- It is important to find out early if a person has HIV. Medicine needs to be taken early. It can keep a person healthy for a longer time.

- Having a sexually transmitted disease (STD) makes it easier to get HIV. People who are sexually active should get tested for STDs every 6 months.

What can I do?

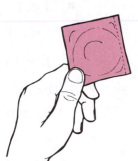

- Teach your teen about HIV and AIDS. Explain why using a condom is so important.

- Encourage your teen to be 100% safe by doing these things:

    - Not having sex (see page 81).

    - Closed mouth kissing.

    - Hugging and rubbing against each other with clothes on.

    - Masturbating alone.

- Teach your teen about safer sex (see page 88).

- Teach your teen to be kind to people who have HIV or AIDS. Tell your teen that he or she will not get AIDS by just being with a person who has AIDS.

- If your teen is sexually active, make sure your teen is tested for STDs every 6 months.

- Get help right away if your teen uses IV drugs. These are drugs that are put into the body using a needle.

When should I get help?

- Your teen has signs of HIV or AIDS (see list on page 99).

- Your teen needs to be tested for HIV or AIDS.

- You are having trouble talking with your teen about HIV. You want someone to talk with your teen.

- Your teen takes IV drugs.

- If you have questions about HIV or AIDS, call AIDS Info at 1-800-448-0440 or the CDC National Prevention Information Network on HIV and AIDS at 1-800-458-5231.

Birth Control

What is it?

Birth control is things people do to prevent getting pregnant. Birth control is also called contraception.

Did you know?

- Not having sex (abstinence) is 100% safe against pregnancy.

- There are a lot of birth control methods that teens can use. They work well if used the right way and every time.

- Without birth control, a girl can get pregnant the first time she has sex. She can get pregnant any time of the month, even during her period.

- Some people think doing these things prevents pregnancy. This is not true. These things should **not be done** to prevent getting pregnant.

  - Standing up after sex.

  - The rhythm method is having unprotected sex on days when a woman is less likely to get pregnant. This is not safe.

  - Pulling out of the vagina before a man comes (ejaculates). Many teens do this. It is not safe.

- Family planning clinics all over the U.S. give birth control to teens.

Birth Control

- Birth control is the duty of both the girl and the boy. They should talk about it before having sex.

- Teens must **always use a condom** along with another form of birth control. Here is a list of birth control methods used by many teens:

Condom or rubber

- Always use a condom even when using other forms of birth control. The condom helps prevent STDs. See page 89 for how to use a condom.

Birth control pill

- It is also called the Pill. It's a very good way to prevent pregnancy.

- A girl must use another form of birth control the first month she starts the Pill.

- A doctor must write an order for birth control pills.

- A girl must not take someone else's pills.

- The Pill must be taken every day, or as told by the doctor.

- If a girl misses taking a pill, she needs to:
  - Take it as soon as she remembers. She can take two pills on the same day.
  - Use another form of birth control until she has her period. She can use spermicides with a condom.

- Some side effects of the Pill are feeling like throwing up, sore breasts, weight gain, headaches, swelling, and light bleeding. These often go away in a few months.

- There are many types of birth control pills. Each has different side effects. The doctor will find the best one for each teen.

- Some teens take the Pill to make their periods regular or for other health reasons.

- Birth control pills don't protect against sexually transmitted diseases (STDs). A condom must be used.

Depo-Provera

- It's a shot that prevents pregnancy for about 12 weeks.

- Side effects are changes in the period, weight gain, and headaches. These often go away in a few months.

- A teen can get the shot at a doctor's office or family planning clinic.

- Depo-Provera does not protect against STDs. A condom must be used.

Diaphragm

- It's a small cup made of soft rubber. A girl puts it in her vagina before sex. It covers the cervix and stops sperm from going into the uterus.

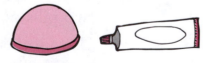

- The diaphragm must be used with a spermicide. Spermicides kill sperm and prevent pregnancy.

- Here's how to use a diaphragm:

Step 1
Put spermicide cream or jelly around the rim and on both sides of the diaphragm.

Step 2
Squeeze the rim of the diaphragm together.

Step 3
Push the diaphragm high up the vagina until it covers the cervix. You can feel the cervix in the middle of the diaphragm.

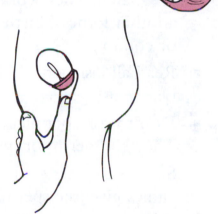

- The diaphragm must be left in the vagina for 8 hours after sex.

- If a girl has sex again during the 8 hours she must put more spermicide into the vagina. The diaphragm needs to be left in place.

- A girl needs to be fitted for a diaphragm at a doctor's office or health clinic. A girl cannot use another girl's diaphragm.

- A girl needs to get a new diaphragm every year. She also needs a new one if she gains or loses more than 10 pounds.

- A diaphragm does not protect against STDs. A condom must also be used.

Spermicides

- They are medicines that are put into the vagina to kill sperm. Spermicides come in many ways (foams, jellies, creams, tablets, suppositories).

- It must be put into the vagina 15 to 20 minutes before sex.

- Spermicides should not be used alone to prevent pregnancy. They work best when used with another form of birth control like the diaphragm or condom.

- Read all instructions that come with spermicides before using.

- Don't wash spermicides out of the vagina after sex. They kill sperm for many hours.

- Spermicides are sold in drugstores. Some health clinics give free spermicides.

- Some people are allergic to spermicides. They get burning in the vagina or penis from spermicides. If allergic, use condoms and lubricants without spermicides.

- Spermicides don't protect against STDs. A condom must be used.

- There are other forms of birth control. They are not used often by teens. They are:
  - Cervical cap
  - Female condom
  - Norplant
  - IUD

- There is a pill that can be taken to stop pregnancy after having sex without birth control. It is called the morning after pill or emergency contraception (EC).
    - It is given:
        - After sex without birth control.
        - In cases of rape.
        - If a condom breaks.
    - It must be taken within 72 hours of unprotected sex.
    - A person can get the morning after pill from a health clinic or a druggist without a doctor's order.
    - The morning after pill does not protect against STDs.

What can I do?

- Learn about birth control methods so you can answer your teen's questions.
- Teach your teen about birth control. Your teen needs to know about birth control even if he or she does not plan to have sex.
- Learning about birth control does not make your teen want to have sex. It helps your teen to make good choices.
- Talk about STDs (see page 93) along with birth control.
- Be open and honest with your teen. Start talking with your teen at a young age.
- Go with your teen to get birth control if she asks you.
- Help your teen choose the best birth control. Help pay for it, if needed. Take your teen to a free clinic for birth control if you can't pay for it.

Birth Control

- Help your teen pick another form of birth control if one method isn't working out.

- Help your teen plan what to say if a partner does not want to use birth control.

- Never tease your teen about birth control. If your teen talks to you about birth control, don't tell anyone. It is private between you and your teen.

- Your teen may get birth control without telling you. If you find out:
  - Stay calm; don't get angry.
  - Don't tell your teen not to use birth control. Your teen may be having sex or thinking about it.
  - Make sure your teen is using birth control the right way.
  - Talk about why it is important to always use condoms.

When should I get help?

- Your teen asks you to go with her to a doctor or clinic to get birth control.

- You think your teen is pregnant.

- You can't talk with your teen about birth control. You want someone to explain it to your teen.

- Your teen won't listen to you.

- Your teen is having sex with many people.

- Your teen uses the morning after pill for birth control.

- Your teen has sex without a condom.

Teen Pregnancy

What is it?

Pregnancy happens when a boy's sperm meets (fertilizes) a girl's egg after sex. The fertilized egg attaches to the wall of the uterus and grows into a baby.

Did you know?

- The U.S. has the highest teen pregnancy rate of most nations.

- 66% of teen mothers are not married.

- Most teen pregnancies are **not** planned.

- A girl can get pregnant the first time she has sex if she does not use birth control. Many teens think this can't happen to them.

- Only 1 in 7 teens gets birth control before starting to have sex. Here are some reasons why:
  - The teen is too shy. She does not want people to know she is having sex.
  - Teen does not know where to get birth control.
  - Teen does not have money to pay for it.
  - Teen does not have a way to get to the doctor, clinic, or store.

Teen Pregnancy

- Some boys feel birth control is the girl's duty. This is not true. It is the duty of both.

- Some teens know about birth control but still get pregnant. Here are some reasons why:
  - They think they won't get pregnant.
  - They didn't plan to have sex.
  - They didn't have birth control with them.
  - One partner does not want to use birth control.

- The first sign of pregnancy is often a missed period. A teen needs to have a pregnancy test if she misses a period and had sex. She can go to a doctor or family planning clinic to be tested. The test at the clinic may be free.

- Other signs of pregnancy are:
  - Feeling sick to the stomach (nausea).
  - Throwing up. This is called morning sickness.
  - Sore breasts.
  - Feeling tired.
  - Gaining weight.

- Prenatal care is the health care a girl needs to have a healthy baby. It is very important to start prenatal care during the first month of pregnancy.

- There are many places to get prenatal care. A teen can go to a doctor's office, or a public health clinic.

- Getting pregnant affects a teen's life forever. Here are some things that can happen:
  - Teen drops out of school.
  - She can't get a good job.
  - She makes very little money.
- Teen fathers also have problems. They often drop out of school.
- Some teens marry because of pregnancy. They have a high breakup rate.
- There are schools and social programs to help teens who are pregnant.

What can I do?

- Begin to talk with your child at an early age about sex. Talk about why it is important to protect against pregnancy and sexually transmitted diseases (STDs).
- Talk with your teen about abstinence (see page 81). Tell your teen they don't need to have sex to fit in or be cool.
- If your teen is having sex, take her to a doctor or clinic for birth control.
- Teach your teen to use birth control **every time** she has sex.
- Talk with your teen about what would happen if she got pregnant (or if he got a girl pregnant). What good things in his or her life would change? What would his or her future look like?

- Know the signs of pregnancy. Take your teen to the doctor if you think she may be pregnant.

- Teach your teen that taking drugs, alcohol, and smoking during pregnancy will hurt the baby.

- A pregnant teen has choices to make. Help your teen to make the right choice. Before she makes a choice, a teen needs to know all her options:

  - **Staying pregnant and keeping the baby.**

    - This choice changes a teen's life forever.

    - The teen needs to know what being a parent means. She needs to know this is forever. She needs to know how much it costs to raise a child and how her life will change.

  - **Ending the pregnancy. This is called abortion.**

    - Abortion is an operation done by a doctor at a clinic or office.

    - Having an abortion can affect a teen's emotions for the rest of her life. No teen should be talked into or out of having an abortion.

    - A teen thinking about abortion can get help at a family planning clinic or other community service agency.

    - Abortion laws vary by state. Most states allow teens to have an abortion without a parent's consent.

    - Public health or family planning clinics can tell a person where to get an abortion.

- **Having the baby and giving the baby up for adoption.**
  - A nurse, doctor, or health clinic can tell a person about adoption and how to do it.
  - Many churches, temples, and community service agencies can help with adoption.
  - The hospital can also help if a teen wants to put her baby up for adoption.
- If your teen is pregnant, help her to have a healthy baby by:
  - Starting prenatal care during the first month of pregnancy.
  - Taking a vitamin daily with at least 600 mcg of folic acid.
  - Staying away from smoking, alcohol, and drugs.
  - Eating right.
  - Staying active.
  - Getting lots of rest.
- At the end of the pregnancy, a teen may have to stop going to school or work. Help your teen do the right things so she has a healthy baby.

When should I get help?

- Your teen started having sex.
- Your teen needs to get birth control.
- You think your teen is pregnant.
- If your pregnant teen uses drugs, alcohol, or smokes, tell the doctor. These things will hurt the baby.

113

- Your teen is pregnant and has these signs:
    - Bleeding
    - Swelling of the face or legs
    - Fast weight gain
    - Bad headaches
    - Trouble peeing
- A new baby needs to go to the doctor for shots and checkups. It is very important to keep all doctor visits.

Masturbation

What is it?

Masturbation is touching one's genitals (privates, sex organs) for sexual pleasure.

Did you know?

- A lot of people masturbate, even married people.
- There is nothing wrong with masturbating. Masturbation does not do bad things to a person.
- Some people are taught to feel guilty about masturbating. This feeling is not healthy.
- Masturbation is a safe form of sex activity. A person cannot get pregnant or an STD from masturbation.
- Masturbation allows a teen to release sexual tension without having sex.
- Two people can touch each other in a sexual way. This is called mutual masturbation.

What can I do?

- Talk to your teen about masturbation. Tell your teen that it is normal.
- Don't make your teen feel guilty about it.
- Tell your teen masturbation is private. It should not be done in public.

When should I get help?

- Your teen is masturbating in public.
- Your teen feels guilty about masturbating or is depressed about it.

Incest

What is it?

Incest is when a family member has sex with or touches in a sexual way another family member. Incest usually involves an adult and a child or teen. Incest is also when a family member makes a child touch them in a sexual way. Family members include parents, grandparents, uncles, aunts, cousins, stepparents, brothers, and sisters.

Did you know?

- Incest is against the law. It must be reported to the police.
- Some things put a family at higher risk for incest such as:
  - Alcohol or drug abuse in adults.
  - Many people living together in a small place.
  - A lot of stress in the family.
  - History of abuse or incest in the family.
- People need outside help to deal with incest.
- Incest can hurt a child for life. The child needs help. He or she needs to talk with a social worker or therapist about what happened.
- Incest can happen to boys and girls at any age.
- Incest is never the child's fault.

Incest

- Many children are afraid to tell anyone what happened because:
    - They think they did something wrong.
    - They think no one will believe them.
    - They were told something bad will happen if they tell anyone.
- Possible signs of incest are:
    - Child knows too much about sex for his or her age.
    - Child always touches his or her genitals.
    - Child acts in a way not normal for age.
    - Child has bad dreams.
    - Child touches other children in a sexual way.
    - Child has a sexually transmitted disease (STD).
    - Child tries to stay away from a certain family member.
    - Child runs away from home.
    - Child has headaches or other problems.
    - Child cries a lot.
- Sometimes sisters and brothers around the same age have sex play. This is common and not harmful when they are very young.

Incest

What can I do?

- Know the signs of incest.

- Talk to your teen about everything.

- Listen to what your teen says. If your teen tells you incest is happening, believe him or her.

- Get help right away if you think your child was abused by a family member. Your child comes first. Don't worry about the family member who is harming your child.

When should I get help?

- You think incest is happening. The entire family may need help. There are many community groups that can help you.

Homosexuality

What is it?

Homosexuality is a strong attraction to people of the same sex. Other words for homosexual are gay and lesbian.

Did you know?

- The cause of homosexuality is not known. Homosexuality is not a disease or mental illness.
- Many homosexuals lead happy lives.
- It is normal for teens to be attracted to teens of the same sex. This can happen during the early teen years. This does not mean the teen is homosexual.
- Teens like to try new things. Some teens have sex play with teens of the same sex. They touch each other's genitals in a sexual way. This does not mean the teens are homosexual.
- A teen may get excited seeing other teens of the same sex in the shower. This does not mean the teen is homosexual.
- Homosexual teens don't choose to be homosexual. They have no control over this.
- When a person says he or she is a homosexual this is called "coming out of the closet."
- Parents of homosexual children often feel anger, guilt, and shame. They wonder what they did wrong.

- It is not a parent's fault if a teen is homosexual. Parents should not blame themselves.

- There are support groups for parents of homosexual children.

- Homosexual teens are often teased by other teens and rejected by their parents. They often have trouble in school. They feel alone. They may drink alcohol or take drugs to try to feel better.

- Homosexual teens are at risk for suicide because they feel alone and different. They are also at risk for violence called gay-bashing.

What can I do?

- Teach your teen to be kind to gay people. Tell your teen homosexuality is not a disease. Talk to your teen about famous gay people like Ellen DeGeneres and Rock Hudson.

- Don't panic if your teen tells you about sex play with a teen of the same sex. This does not mean your teen is homosexual. He or she may just be trying new things.

- Don't blame yourself if your teen is homosexual. There is nothing you did wrong.

- Don't be angry if you find out your teen is homosexual. Stay calm. Your teen needs your love and support.

- Don't try to talk your teen out of being a homosexual. Don't tell your teen this is a passing phase.

- Don't put your teen down or tease your teen.

- Help your teen find friends who support him or her.

- Join a support group for parents of homosexual children. Talking with other parents will help you give your teen love and support.

When should I get help?

- Your teen is troubled by his or her feelings for teens of the same sex.
- You have trouble accepting that your teen is homosexual.

Teen Safety 5

Notes

_____

_____

_____

_____

_____

_____

_____

_____

_____

_____

_____

_____

_____

Driving

What is it?

Teen gets a driver's license and
drives a car or motorcycle.
In most states teens can get
a driver's license at age 16.
In some states, the age is 18.

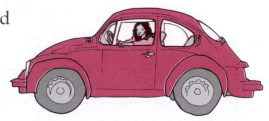

Did you know?

- Teens want to drive. It gives them freedom. It makes them feel grown up.

- Car accidents are the number 1 killer of teens in the U.S.

- Some teens don't wear seat belts.

- Some teens take risks when they drive. Teens don't see risks on the road like a long time driver. Teens may be looking around instead of watching the road. This can lead to crashes.

- Drunk driving can kill. No one should drive after drinking alcohol or taking drugs. No one should ride in a car if the driver has been drinking or taking drugs.

- In many states, teens lose their license if they drink and drive. This happens the first time a teen is caught.

- Insurance rates are much higher for teens. Most insurance companies give discounts to teens that have good school grades.

Driving

- Many high schools offer driving classes. This is a good way for teens to learn to drive. Teens need a lot of practice driving.

- Sometimes teens drive with too many people in the car. This is not safe. Driving alone is safer than with a group of friends. Friends can take a teen's mind off the road.

- Loud music in the car can take a teen's mind off the road.

- Driving in bad weather or at night is harder.

- Teens need to know what to do if an accident happens.

What can I do?

- Help your teen learn to drive. Let your teen drive with you in the car. Make sure your teen is a safe driver.

- Get your teen to take driving lessons.

- Teach your teen not to use a cell phone or eat food while driving.

- Set driving rules for your teen like:
  - Never drink and drive.
  - Never take drugs and drive.
  - Never ride in a car if the driver drank alcohol or took drugs.
  - Always wear a seat belt, even in the back seat.
  - Never take more people in the car than there are seat belts. Everyone in the car must wear a seat belt.

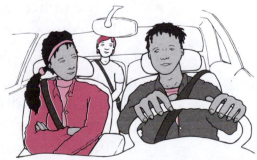

- Always take money with you to call home or take a bus.

- Never let another person drive your car.

- Drive on main streets. Stay off back roads.

- Don't drive when you are tired. If you are sleepy, pull over and call home.

- Don't pick up anyone you don't know.

- Find your keys before you walk to the car. Get in the car right away and lock all the doors.

- Never take a ride from a stranger if your car breaks down.

- Set a time for your teen to be home. Have your teen call home if he or she will be late.

- Shop around for car insurance to get the best price.

- Decide who pays for insurance, gas, tickets, and repairs.

- If your teen buys an old car, help fix it up. Make sure it is safe.

- Teach your teen what to do if he or she gets a flat tire.

- If your teen is in a car crash, tell him or her to:

  - Call 911 if anyone is hurt.

  - Call the police. Stay with the car until the police comes.

  - Get the name, phone number, address, license plate number, driver's license number, and insurance company of the other cars in the accident.

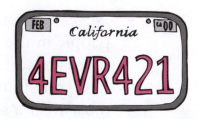

- Get the name and phone number of everyone who saw the crash.
- Write down everything about the crash.
- Report the crash to your insurance company. Do this even if it is not your fault.
- Save names, numbers, and anything else from the crash.
- Get a copy of the police report.
- Always tell your parents.

- Keep a flashlight and first-aid kit in the car.

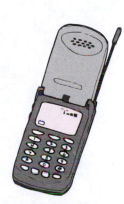

- You may want your teen to have a cell phone in the car to call for help.
- If your teen drinks and drives, take away his or her license.
- If your teen gets speeding tickets or comes home too late don't let your teen drive for a month.
- Go over these things with your teen before you let your teen drive alone:
  - The dangers of alcohol and driving.
  - What to do if teen drinks alcohol and has the car.
  - What to do in a car crash.
  - Driving in bad weather or at night.
  - What to do if the car breaks down.
  - What will happen if your teen breaks one of your rules.
- Always know where your teen is going and when he or she will be back.

Driving

When should I get help?

- Your teen had a crash and did not report it.
- Your teen is drinking or taking drugs and driving.
- Your teen keeps getting tickets.
- Your teen does not listen to you but needs to drive because of work or school.

Alcohol

What is it?

Alcohol is a liquid people drink that can make them high and act silly. This is called being drunk or intoxicated. Alcohol is sometimes called booze.

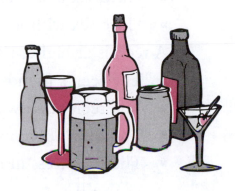

Did you know?

- Many parents don't know the dangers of alcohol. They think drinking alcohol is not as bad as taking drugs.

- By age 13, 1 in 4 teens drinks alcohol.

- Drinking may be a sign that a teen has other problems. Teens with low self-esteem often drink alcohol to feel better.

- Drinking alcohol is bad for a teen's brain. It can harm for life a teen's ability to think and learn.

- The leading cause of teen deaths is car accidents in which one driver was drunk. No one should drink alcohol and drive.

- It is never too early to tell kids why drinking is bad. Some kids start to drink alcohol as young as 9.

- A teen can become an alcoholic. This can happen **without** the parents knowing it.

Alcohol

- Teens who drink are more likely to:
  - Do poorly in school.
  - Drop out of school.
  - Have sex at an earlier age.
  - Have sex without a condom.
- A teen is at higher risk of drinking alcohol if:
  - The teen's friends drink alcohol.
  - The teen has low self-esteem.
  - The teen's parents or older brothers or sisters drink.
  - There is stress in the home from divorce, illness, or death.
- Some teens drink 5 or more drinks at a time. This is called binge drinking. Some teens die from binge drinking.
- Some drinks have more alcohol than others. Some fruit flavored wines have 20% alcohol. The wine tastes sweet. Teens may not know the drink has so much alcohol.
- A teen can get drunk after one drink. This can happen with wine, beer, or other alcohol.
- Some teens drink alcohol that is in the home. They often add water to the bottle to replace what they drank.
- Safe use of alcohol must be learned. Teens watch how their parents use alcohol. They copy that example.
- A person who sells or gives alcohol to someone under the drinking age is breaking the law. That person can go to jail.

Alcohol

- The legal age for drinking is 21.
- If you give alcohol to a person under age and something bad happens, it is your fault.
- Some teens drink after school if they are alone and bored.
- Many teens drink to be cool or to fit in. Alcohol helps a teen feel less shy. Some teens drink when they are upset.
- There are groups such as Alcoholics Anonymous (called AA) that help teens stop using alcohol.
- Some teens need to go to a hospital to stop drinking alcohol.

What can I do?

- Talk with your teen about the bad things that can come from drinking alcohol.
- Tell your teen that people die from binge drinking.
- Tell your teen he or she does not need to drink alcohol to fit in.
- Teach your teen that alcohol is bad for the growing brain. Alcohol can harm them for life.
- Teach your teen safe rules about alcohol:
  - Alcohol is bad for teens.
  - Never drive after drinking alcohol.
  - Never let anyone drive after drinking alcohol.
  - Don't drink when you are alone.
  - Never drink to get drunk.

- ■ Don't drink to feel better. Alcohol does not fix problems.

- ■ Don't drink if you are depressed or angry.

- Teach your teen to decide who will drive when going out with friends. This person must not drink **any** alcohol. He or she is called the designated driver.

- Teach your teen never to get into a car if the driver drank alcohol. Make sure your teen knows to call you for a ride. Always be ready to go get your teen.

- Tell your teen to bring money when going out. Your teen can call home or take a bus or taxi if there is a problem.

- Don't fight with your teen if he or she is drunk. Don't let your teen go to sleep if he or she is drunk. Your teen can slip into a coma and die. Walk with your teen until the alcohol gets out of the body.

- Help your teen find things to do after school. Try to be there when your teen comes home from school. Know what your teen is doing after school.

- Watch for signs that your teen is drinking such as:
  - ■ Acting silly.
  - ■ Mood swings.
  - ■ Change in friends.

- Lying.
- Smell of alcohol on your teen's breath.
- Alcohol is missing from the home.
- Get your teen into a group like AA if he or she drinks alcohol.

When should I get help?

- You think your teen is drinking.
- Call 911 if your teen is hard to wake up after drinking.

Drugs

What is it?

Something a person eats, smokes, or injects to feel good or get high.

Did you know?

- Drugs are everywhere. Kids as young as 8 or 9 use drugs. It is never too early to start talking with kids about why drugs are bad.
- A teen can die from using drugs one time.
- Teens start using drugs for many reasons such as:
  - They want to try something new.
  - They want to fit in.
  - To feel better about themselves.
  - To escape problems at home or school.
- At first teens take drugs to feel good. This is called getting high. Later they need drugs to stop feeling bad. This is called drug addiction.
- Teens can become addicted in a short time. Parents often don't know that their teen is taking drugs.
- Here are some signs that a teen may be using drugs:
  - Drop in school grades.
  - Teen skips classes or stops going to school.
  - Lying and stealing.

Drugs

- Money and other things are missing from the home.
- Teen is alone most of the time.
- Change in eating habits.
- Big change in mood.
- Fighting with friends and family.
- Violent moments.
- Glassy eyes.
- Slurred speech.
- Getting sick a lot.
- Teen can't get up in the morning.
- Drugs found in teen's room.
- Smell of drugs like marijuana.
- Teen is spending money very fast.

- Parents may be too busy to see the signs. They may think it can't happen to them. Drug use can happen to anyone.

- Drugs are bad for the brain. They can harm for life how a person thinks and acts.

- There are many drugs. Here are the most common ones:

  - **Marijuana**

    Other names for marijuana are pot, weed, grass, joint, and roach. It is the most common drug. It is smoked.

  - **Cocaine**

    Other names are coke, snow, and flake. It is snorted into the nose.

Drugs

- **Crack cocaine**

  Other names are crack, freebase rocks, and rock cocaine. This drug is smoked.

- **LSD**

  This drug is also called acid. It is taken by mouth.

- **PCP**

  Other names are angel dust, wack, and loveboat. It is taken by mouth.

- **Speed**

  Other names are amphetamines, black beauties, and hearts. There are many types of speed. It can be taken by mouth, smoked, snorted, or injected.

- **Heroin**

  Other names are smack and horse. It is injected into a vein.

- **Methamphetamine**

  Other names are ice, crank, meth, and crystal. It comes in a crystal or powder form. It is taken by mouth.

- **Inhalants**

  These are things that teens breathe in (sniff) to get high. Sniffing fumes is called huffing. Some things teens sniff are glue, gasoline, and aerosol cans like those from paint and whipped cream.

- **Designer drugs**

  Other names are MDA, MMDA, MDM, and MDE. Each one of these drugs is different. They are taken mostly by mouth.

What can I do?

- Start talking with your child early about why drugs are bad. Talk about all the bad things that can come from taking drugs.

- Teach your child to say **NO** to drugs. Say this over and over again. Make it clear to your child that drugs are bad.

- Tell your teen that someone can put a drug into his or her drink. Your teen should never walk away from their drink.

- Teens who take drugs often have other problems. Listen to what your teen says to you. Help your teen. If you do not know what to do, get outside help.

- Watch for signs that your teen may be taking drugs (see pages 134–135).

- Watch for signs that your teen may be huffing. Some things to look for are:

  - Sores or rash near nose and mouth.

  - Paint on face or clothes.

  - Smell of chemicals on clothes or in teen's room.

  - Red eyes.

  - Runny nose.

  - Unsteady walk.

- Help your teen find things to do after school. Know what your teen does after school. Check to see if your teen is doing the things he or she says they are doing. Don't leave your teen alone a lot.

- Get to know your teen's friends. Help your teen pick good friends.
- Get your teen into sports or other good groups like boys and girls clubs.
- If you find drugs in your teen's room, take action right away. Your teen can die from taking drugs. Talk to your teen about what you found. Get outside help right away.
- Talk honestly with your teen if other members of the family have a problem with drugs. Talk about addiction. Talk about how hard it is to stop taking drugs. Talk about how drugs ruin people's lives.

When should I get help?

- Get help right away if you think your teen is taking drugs.

Smoking

What is it?

It is breathing smoke from a cigarette into the lungs. It is a bad habit. It costs a lot of money. It makes people sick. People die from smoking.

Did you know?

- Children as young as 8 try smoking.
- About 1 in 3 teens who try smoking becomes a steady smoker.
- Smoking is like a drug. Once you start, it is very hard to stop.
- Some kids chew tobacco (called snuff). This is just as bad as smoking. It can cause mouth and throat cancer. It can also cause tooth loss and gum disease.
- Teens smoke for many reasons such as:
  - They want to look cool.
  - They want to look or feel grown-up.
  - Someone smokes at home.
  - Their friends smoke.
  - They are bored.
  - They are hungry or they want to lose weight.
  - Stress at home or school.

- They want to know what it's like to smoke.
- They see people smoke in the movies and on TV.

What can I do?

- Start talking with your child early about why smoking is bad.
- Some things you can tell your child are:
  - Once you start smoking, it's very hard to stop.
  - It costs a lot of money. You can save about $70 a month by not smoking.
  - It gives you bad breath and makes your teeth yellow.
  - No one wants to kiss a smoker.
  - Smoking causes cancer. It makes your heart and lungs sick.
  - Smoking makes you do poorly in sports. It makes it harder for you to breathe.
  - You may get kicked out of school if you are caught smoking.
- Teach your teen to like him or herself. Tell your teen he or she does not need to smoke to fit in or look cool.
- Teens learn by example. If you smoke, your teen will also smoke. This may be a good time for you to stop smoking. Get your family to help you stop. Let your teen see how hard it is to stop.
- Get your teen involved in sports, band, or other things that don't allow smoking.

Smoking

- Help your teen plan how to say **NO** when friends want him or her to smoke. Here are some things to say:
  - No thanks, I like myself too much to smoke.
  - My coach will kick me off the team if he catches me smoking.
  - I will be grounded for a month if my parents catch me.
  - My parents will not let me use the car if I smoke.
- Encourage your teen to be with friends that don't smoke.
- Look for signs that your teen smokes:
  - Cigarette butts in pockets.
  - Yellow fingers.
  - Hair and clothes smell of smoke.
- Do these things if your teen smokes:
  - Talk with your teen's teacher about a school project on why smoking is bad. Your teen might stop smoking from what he or she learns.
  - Promise to buy your teen something if he or she stops smoking for 1 month.
  - Call the American Lung Association at 1-800-586-4872. They can help you find help for your teen.
  - Ask your teen's school about a program to help your teen stop smoking.

■ Talk with your teen's coach or counselor about other things to try.

When should I get help?

- Your teen smokes.
- You think your teen is smoking.

Body Piercing

What is it?

Body piercing is making holes in the skin for rings or studs.

Did you know?

- Many teens have their bodies pierced. Common places are the earlobes, eyebrow, belly button, and tongue.

- Teens get pierced because they think it looks good. They want people to see them and talk about it.

- Some teens get too many piercings. This can be a sign of other problems.

- Teens can get infection, hepatitis B & C, and tetanus from body piercing. These are very serious diseases.

- Some teens use a sewing needle from home to make a hole in the skin. This can cause infection. Some signs of infection are:
    - Redness around the hole.
    - Red streaks on the skin.
    - Yellow liquid (pus) oozing from hole.
    - Swelling.
    - Pain.

Body Piercing

- Some places use a machine called a piercing gun. It is hard to clean. It is safe only for piercing the earlobe.

- People can get disease and infection from the tool or needle used for piercing. New needles or clean (sterile) tools must be used each time. New latex gloves need to be worn each time.

- Some states have laws for body piercing.

- No one high on drugs or alcohol should get a piercing. They may not know what they are doing.

- Belly-button piercing takes up to a year to heal. A teen can get a very bad infection.

What can I do?

- Tell your teen that piercing can make him or her sick.

- If your teen wants to get pierced, have your teen wait 2 months before getting pierced. Tell your teen to take time to think about it.

- If your teen is sure about getting pierced, help your teen pick a safe place to have it done. Make sure your teen has his or her shots for hepatitis and tetanus.

- Don't get upset if your teen gets pierced. Help your teen stop at one piercing.

Body Piercing

When should I get help?

- Your teen insists on getting body piercing. Find a safe place for your teen.

- Your teen has signs of infection like redness, pus, heat, and pain.

- Your teen has more than 2 body piercings.

Tattoos

What is it?

Tattoos are marks or designs in the skin that don't come off. They are made by drawing on the skin with needles. Tattoos stay on the skin forever.

Did you know?

- Many people get tattoos. It does not mean they are bad or in a gang.

- It is very hard to get rid of a tattoo. It costs a lot of money. Some of the tattoo may not come off.

- Some teens pick a design that is not right for an adult. A teen will be stuck with the tattoo for life.

- Many adults wish they did not get a tattoo when they were a teen.

- A person can get infections, hepatitis B or C, and other diseases from getting a tattoo.

- People high on drugs or alcohol should not get a tattoo. They may not know what they are doing.

- Some states have laws for safe tattoos. People should only go to legal tattoo places.

- In many states, teens under 18 need a parent's OK to get tattoos. Many teens sign their mom's or dad's name. They are breaking the law.

What can I do?

- If your teen wants a tattoo make sure your teen knows that tattoos don't come off easily. Have your teen talk to a doctor about how hard it is to take off a tattoo.

- Talk to your teen about other ways to look cool like hair color and style.

- Learn about the laws of your state. Make sure your teen knows the law.

- Ask your teen to wait 1 or 2 months before getting a tattoo. Your teen should think it over. A tattoo is forever. Will your teen want it in 10 years?

- Have your teen talk to people who wish they did not get a tattoo.

- If your teen is certain about getting a tattoo, help your teen pick a good design. Have the tattoo put where it can be covered with clothes.

- Have the tattoo done at a safe and legal place.

- Make sure your teen has his or her shots for hepatitis and tetanus.

- If your teen gets a tattoo, don't get too upset. Help your teen to stop at one tattoo.

When should I get help?

- Your teen wants a tattoo. You want to find a safe and legal place.

- Your teen got a tattoo. The skin shows signs of infection like redness, pus and heat.

Gangs

What is it?

A gang is a group of teens who have rules and a leader. They hang out together. They look the same. They dress in gang colors. They fight other gangs and break the law.

Did you know?

- Gangs are everywhere. More boys than girls are in gangs. Most teens in gangs are between the ages of 12 and 17.

- Many gangs use drugs, steal, and break the law in other ways.

- Teens in gangs are violent. Sometimes they use guns.

- Many teens die or are badly hurt in gangs.

- Teens join gangs because:
  - They want to fit in.
  - They want love and support.
  - They think it's cool to be in a gang.
  - They want to feel a part of something.

- Teens who are close to their family usually don't join gangs. They don't need gangs for love and support.

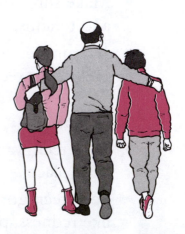

What can I do?

- Ask your teen what he thinks about gangs. Talk about why gangs are bad.

- Ask yourself if you spend enough time with your teen. Many teens are alone too much. They get into gangs because they have nothing to do.

- Spend time together as a family. Start a family project. Do a sport as a family.

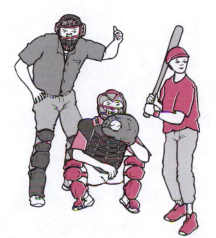

- Teens need other teens. Help your teen find safe clubs to join. Some clubs are the YMCA, church groups, sports teams, and school clubs.

- Talk to the school or police about gangs in your area. Find out what you can do.

- Watch how your teen dresses. Don't let your teen wear gang colors. He can be hurt or killed.

When should I get help?

- Your teen is in a gang.
- You are worried your teen will join a gang.
- Your teen is bullied by a gang.
- Your teen feels pressure to join a gang.

Word List

A

- **abortion**—An operation done by a doctor to end a pregnancy.
- **abstinence**—Not having sex.
- **addiction**—A strong need or desire to do something like smoke or take drugs.
- **adoption**—To give a child to another family, or take a child into your family.
- **alcoholic**—A person who cannot control how much alcohol he or she drinks.
- **Alcoholics Anonymous (AA)**—A group that helps people stop drinking alcohol.
- **allowance**—Money given to someone at regular intervals.
- **anal sex**—Putting the penis into the anus.
- **anus**—Another word for rectum.
- **appetite**—A normal desire for food.

B

- **binge eating**—Eating large amounts of food in a short time.
- **birth control**—Things people do to prevent getting pregnant.
- **booze**—A slang word for drinks that have alcohol in them.
- **Boys and Girls Club**—A place to go in the neighborhood that has activities for children.

- **breast**—Part of the chest. In women, breast glands make milk after childbirth.
- **bully**—Someone who picks on or tries to start a fight with smaller or weaker people.

C

- **cervix**—The opening of the uterus into the vagina.
- **cigarette**—Tobacco rolled in paper for smoking. People who smoke can get addicted. Smoking causes cancer and many other diseases.
- **circumcision**—An operation to remove the foreskin around the penis.
- **chores**—Things that people must do around the house.
- **coitus**—Putting the penis into the vagina.
- **coma**—A deep sleep-like state caused by sickness or injury.
- **condom**—A latex cover put on a hard penis before sex. It prevents pregnancy and many sexually transmitted diseases.
- **contraception**—Another word for birth control.
- **copulation**—Another word for sex.
- **curfew**—The time a person needs to be home.

D

- **deodorant**—A spray, cream, or other substance put on the body to stop bad body smell.
- **designated driver**—A person who does not drink alcohol so he or she can drive other people home.
- **drinking**—A word used to mean drinking liquids that have alcohol.

Word List

E

- **ejaculate**—When semen comes out of the penis during orgasm.
- **erection**—A hard penis.

F

- **foreskin**—Loose skin around the tip of the penis. It can be removed by an operation called circumcision.

G

- **gay**—Having a strong attraction to people of the same sex.
- **gay bashing**—Making fun of or hurting someone because he or she is gay.
- **genitals**—Parts of the body used in sex.
- **grounding**—A type of punishment that does not allow a teen to go out with friends for a period of time.

H

- **hormones**—Chemicals made in the body to do certain things.
- **huffing**—Breathing or sniffing fumes from glue or aerosol cans to get high.

I

- **inebriated**—Another word for being drunk.
- **infection**—Sickness caused by germs you cannot see. An infection can happen inside the body or on the skin. Signs of skin infection are redness, heat, pain, and liquid or pus oozing from the skin.
- **intoxicated**—Another word for being drunk.

Word List

L

- **laxative**—Medicine taken to help a person have a BM or bowel movement.
- **learning disability**—Trouble reading and learning.
- **lesbian**—A girl who is attracted to other girls.
- **library**—A place where books are kept. People go to the library to read books or to take books home for a period of time.

O

- **oral sex**—The act of putting the mouth on the penis or the vagina.
- **orgasm**—Another word for climax.
- **ovulation**—When an egg comes out of a woman's ovary. She can get pregnant at this time if she has sex without using birth control.

P

- **peer pressure**—When friends try to get a person to do something.
- **period**—The bloody discharge that comes out of a girl's vagina each month. This is called menstruation.
- **prenatal**—The time before childbirth when a woman is expecting a baby.
- **puberty**—The time of fast growth when boys' and girls' bodies change from that of a child to an adult.
- **punishment**—A penalty given to a person for doing something wrong.

Word List

- **pus**—A thick liquid that comes out of the body when there is an infection. The liquid is usually yellow or green and can smell bad.

R

- **rape**—Forcing someone to have sex.

S

- **scrotum**—The pouch or sac on the outside of a man's body behind the penis that holds the testicles.
- **semen**—Thick white fluid that comes out the penis during ejaculation.
- **sperm**—The man's seed. Sperm combine with the woman's egg to make a baby.
- **spermicide**—A cream or foam that kills sperm.
- **steroid**—Drugs taken by people to get stronger and do better in sports. Steroids are sometimes ordered by doctors for certain diseases.

T

- **teen years**—In this book, the teen years refer to ages 9–19 years.
- **testicles**—The part of the man's body that makes sperm.
- **tutors**—Special teachers to help people with school work or to learn certain things.

W

- **wet dream**—Ejaculation during sleep.

What's in This Book from A to Z

What's in This Book from A to Z

What's in This Book from A to Z

What's in This Book from A to Z

What's in This Book from A to Z

People We Want to Thank

We want to thank the following people for their help with this book:

Albert Barnett, MD

Art Brown, BA, MA

Diane Brown, MPH

Frank J. Brown, BS, MBA

Angelique Maree Crain, AB, MA

Robert Cummings, MD, Ph.D.

Gene Getz Jr

Michelle Getz

JoAnn Heller

Judi Leonard, MSN, PNP, CS

Shanine Jackson

Kimberly Mayer, BA

Thomas R. Mayer, MD

Hannah Lee

Nancy L. McDade

Ruby Raya-Morones, MD

Mona Moreno

Richard C. Palmer, MD

Greg Perez, BS

Kemy Pyper

Gary Richwald, MD, MPH

Steven Rosenberg, MD

Nancy Rushton, RN, BSN

Michael Satin

Andrew Scott, BA, B.ed

Emily Scott, B.ed

Jennifer Ann Scott

Jane Song

Benz Teeranitayatarn

Dylann Tharp

Irene Verdi

Camille Wall, MSW, LCSW

Vivian Wilson

Other Books in the Series

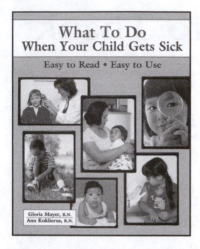

ISBN 978-0-9701245-0-0
$12.95

What To Do
When Your Child Gets Sick*

There are many things you can do at home for your child. At last, an easy to read, easy to use book written by two nurses who know. This book tells you:

- What to look for when your child is sick.
- When to call the doctor.
- How to take your child's temperature.
- What to do when your child has the flu.
- How to care for cuts and scrapes.
- What to feed your child when he or she is sick.
- How to stop the spread of infection.
- How to prevent accidents around your home.
- What to do in an emergency.

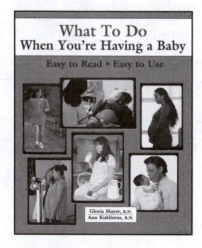

ISBN 978-0-9701245-6-2
$12.95

What To Do
When You're Having a Baby

There are many things a woman can do to have a healthy baby. Here's an easy to read, easy to use book written by two nurses that tells you:

- How to get ready for pregnancy.
- About the health care you need during pregnancy.
- Things you should not do when you are pregnant.
- How to take care of yourself so you have a healthy baby.
- Body changes you have each month.
- Simple things you can do to feel better.
- Warning signs of problems and what to do about them.
- All about labor and delivery.
- How to feed and care for your new baby.

Also available in Spanish.
***Also available in Vietnamese, Chinese and Korean.**
To order, call (800) 434-4633.

Other Books in the Series

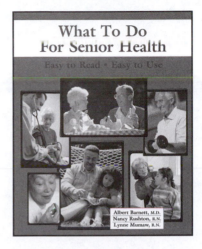

ISBN 978-0-9701245-4-8
$12.95

What To Do
For Senior Health*

There are many things that you can do to take charge of your health during your senior years. This book tells about:

- Body changes that come with aging.
- Common health problems of seniors.
- Things to consider about health insurance.
- How to choose a doctor and where to get health care.
- Buying and taking medicines.
- Simple things you can do to prevent falls and accidents.
- What you can do to stay healthy.

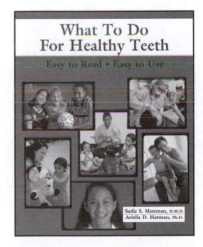

ISBN 978-0-9720148-0-9
$12.95

What To Do
For Healthy Teeth

It is important to take good care of your teeth from an early age. This book tells how to do that. It also explains all about teeth, gums, and how dentists work with you to keep your teeth healthy.

- How to care for your teeth and gums.
- What you need to care for your teeth and gums.
- Caring for your teeth when you're having a baby.
- Caring for your child's teeth.
- When to call the dentist.
- What to expect at a dental visit.
- Dental care needs for seniors.
- What to do if you hurt your mouth or teeth.

Also available in Spanish.
*Also available in Vietnamese.
To order, call (800) 434-4633.